Healthcare Quality and Performance Improvement Case Studies

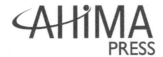

AHIMA PRESS

ISBN: **978-1-58426-919-9**
eISBN: **978-1-58426-920-5**
AHIMA Product No.: AB112722

AHIMA Staff:
Sarah Cybulski, MA, Assistant Editor
Megan Grennan, Director, Content Production and AHIMA Press
James Pinnick, Vice President, Content and Learning Solutions
Christine Scheid, Content Development Manager
Rachel Schratz, MA, Associate Digital Content Developer

Cover image: © Melissa Welch

For more information, including updates, about AHIMA Press publications, visit **http://www.ahima.org /education/press.**

American Health Information Management Association
233 North Michigan Avenue, 21st Floor
Chicago, Illinois 60601-5809
ahima.org

Healthcare Quality and Performance Improvement Case Studies

Patrice L. Spath, MA, RHIT

2023

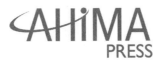

Contents

Detailed Contents

About the Author

Patrice L. Spath, MA, RHIT, is a health information management professional with broad experience in healthcare quality and safety improvement. She is president of Brown-Spath & Associates (www.brownspath.com), a healthcare publishing and training company based in Forest Grove, Oregon. During the past 45 years, Patrice has presented more than 400 educational programs on healthcare quality management topics and has completed numerous quality and patient safety program consultations for healthcare organizations.

Ms. Spath has authored and edited many books, book chapters, and peer-reviewed articles for Health Administration Press, Health Forum/AHA Press, Jossey-Bass, OR Manager, Brown-Spath & Associates, and other groups. Her recent books include *Introduction to Healthcare Quality Management*, 4th ed. (Health Administration Press, 2023); *Applying Quality Management in Healthcare: A Systems Approach*, 5th ed. (Health Administration Press, 2022); *Strategic Management of Health Care Organizations*, 3rd ed. (Zovio, Inc., 2022); *Fundamentals of Health Care Quality Management*, 5th ed. (Brown-Spath & Associates, 2019); and *Error Reduction in Health Care*, 2nd ed. (Jossey-Bass, 2011).

Since 2004 Ms. Spath has taught undergraduate and graduate online courses on healthcare quality management and patient safety at several schools, including the University of Alabama in Birmingham, Oregon Health & Science University, Missouri Western State University in St. Joseph, Pacific University in Forest Grove, OR and Drexel University College of Medicine, Philadelphia, PA.

Ms. Spath is a member of the American Health Information Management Association (AHIMA) and has been a member of the Council on Certification, Council on Accreditation and co-chair of the Data Governance & Analytics Practice Council. In 2020 she received the AHIMA Distinguished Member Award. In 1987 Patrice served on the board of the National Association of Health Quality (NAHQ) and was a member of the 1982 NAHQ group that developed the Certified Professional in Healthcare Quality (CPHQ) exam.

Preface

To achieve high quality healthcare services, organizations have a systematic quality and performance improvement process. This process is known as quality management, which is a way of doing business that continuously improves services to achieve better performance.

Healthcare organizations keep track of performance through various measurement activities. The purpose of measurement is to provide information about the quality of patient care and healthcare support functions. Measurement results are evaluated to determine how well the organization is performing and the measurement data are compared to performance expectations. If expectations are met, performance continues to be measured and periodically assessed. If expectations are not met, performance gaps are investigated, and changes are made to achieve better performance. Quality management never reaches an endpoint. Performance continues to be evaluated through ongoing measurement activities.

To effectively support quality management activities, healthcare professionals must know how to gather valid measurement data and understand how to analyze measurement data to identify improvement opportunities. And they must know how to make process changes that will correct undesirable performance. The case studies in this workbook are designed to provide students an opportunity to apply the tools and techniques necessary to effectively support quality and performance improvement in healthcare. The case studies portray situations faced by quality professionals, unit managers, and front-line staff in a variety of healthcare settings.

Each case study includes a description, instructions, and some have helpful tips. Diagrams, figures, case scenarios and other support materials are provided when necessary to complete a case study. Some case studies are accompanied by blank answer sheets (Word™ files) or data sets (Excel™ files). These can be downloaded from the AHIMA student website (http://ahimapress.org/Spath9199/). You can modify them as needed to complete the case studies.

The case studies are organized into general categories that correspond to the chapters in the book *Quality and Performance Improvement in Healthcare*, however, it is not necessary to have this book to complete the case studies. Your instructor may adjust the sequencing of the case studies to meet the curriculum requirements of your program. In addition, your instructor may modify some cases or choose to use some for in-class discussion rather than assign them as independent work.

Acknowledgments

AHIMA Press would like to thank Anissa McBreen, RHIA, and Lynn Ward, EdD, RHIA, CPHIMS, for their technical review of this textbook.

This case study book has greatly benefited from the experiences of instructors and students. Their contributions are appreciated.

Foreword

Quality is everyone's business and everyone's responsibility. Quality management in healthcare is the effort we make to continuously improve our ability to meet or exceed our customers' needs and expectations. The reason the definition is not confined merely to customer needs is that the customer does not always know what they need. When patients come to a healthcare provider to be treated, they do not always know the treatments they may need or what type of care to expect.

How do organizations and departments within those organizations achieve quality? Achieving quality requires knowledge of customer expectations, knowledge of output and process performance, and management of employee actions to continuously improve the processes. The first step is identify your customer. The customer is:

- The one you serve
- The one that receives the benefit of your labor
- The reason you have a job.

Healthcare organizations need to consider both external and internal customers. We must stop thinking of ourselves as isolated departments competing against each other. We must reward people for working together to achieve better results. For instance, if the hospital physical therapy department struggles with CPT codes for billing, the health information management (HIM) department should offer help. For many, it is easy to identify external customers, as they are the people we serve when we perform our daily job duties. Your internal customers are the departments and individuals receiving the benefit of your work efforts.

Once you identify your internal and external customers, the next step is to evaluate how well you meet these customers' expectations. The first thing you need to do is set up a dialogue with them. Do not just mail out a survey – talk to them. Take the time to periodically sit down with your customers and discuss their needs and expectations. They will tell you their expectations and it is your responsibility to understand their needs if they do not. It is important to understand more about each other's job. Break down the barriers and start connecting and communicating with one another. Everyone involved in healthcare is part of one big process and we should understand our interconnectedness. We cannot perform activities in isolation; we are part of a whole.

After identifying and learning more about your customers, the next step is to measure your output performance. If you do not measure baseline performance, you cannot know how you have improved. Once you measure your performance you need to identify the critical processes which impact the outputs (your service). Identifying which processes impact your outputs allows you to continually improve those processes; however, an inspection system that just measures output does not tell you *why* you have bad output. Inspection alone does not build quality. We need to reflect on how we do what we do and find ways to continually improve.

We should focus on three parts of process: output, input, and actions. Output is affected by input and actions. If you only focus on output, you only know what is good and what is bad. Output only tells you, for example, what your patient complication rate is. Patient complication rate is only raw data because you don't know why the rate is what it is. If the normal rate for complications is approximately five percent, you may be satisfied. Only until your facility's complication rate exceeds five percent do you become concerned. However, when we set a standard (for example, no more than five percent complication rate) and reach it, most people think they have succeeded. But this is not quality improvement. We should always strive for continual improvement.

When you only have an inspection system and you expect that system to improve quality you will not see results. Often this system motivates a healthcare facility to squeeze in evaluative efforts and improvements in just the few months immediately preceding a Joint Commission survey. Once you pass the survey and get accredited for three years, then what do you do? You wait until the next inspection. An inspection system alone does not help improve quality overall in the long term.

One mistake that has been made in the past is that quality management has been the job of the quality management (QM) coordinator. What happens is that the managers and physicians turn the responsibility of quality over to the coordinator. The QM coordinator can provide data on output and tell other managers and physicians how they are doing in certain areas, but she cannot personally improve processes. Rather, everyone in the organization must participate. The people that work in the processes often have the greatest knowledge to contribute because of their background and experience. The hospital admissions clerk who has been working in admissions for fifteen years has the equivalent of an MBA in patient admissions. We need her knowledge to improve the process. Managers simply cannot have all the information that is needed to improve performance.

There is variation in every healthcare process. If you carefully examined every process, you would find tremendous quality improvement potentials. To change inadequate and ineffectual work activities, you must find systematic ways to go through your department's processes. When you look at your processes more carefully, you will find all kinds of variation. Reducing the variations that occur when different employees perform tasks will eliminate a lot of waste and error within the processes. Once the most efficient process is defined, you need to measure the process itself. To gain control of the process do not just measure output (the outcome), but also measure compliance with the individual process steps.

In this case study workbook, you learn how to measure, evaluate and improve healthcare performance using a variety of quality management tools and techniques. Quality and performance improvement continues to be a high priority in all healthcare settings.

Online Resources

For Students

Student worksheets are available online to accompany this textbook. Visit http://www.ahimapress.org /Spath9199/ and register your unique student access code that is provided inside the front cover of this textbook to download the files.

For Instructors

Instructor materials for this book are provided only to approved educators. Materials include case study answers, instructional tips, and resources. Please visit http://www.ahima.org/publications/educators .aspx for further instruction. If you have any questions regarding the instructor materials, please contact AHIMA Customer Relations at (800) 335-5535 or submit a customer support request at https:// my.ahima.org/messages.

Introduction and History of Performance Improvement

1

1.1 Factors that Inhibit Improvements in Healthcare

Description

Despite advances in medical technology and research in recent years, the quality of healthcare is not what it could be. In this project you'll learn about historical and current factors that inhibit healthcare improvements.

Instructions

1. Read the article: D.M. Berwick. "Improvement, Trust, and the Healthcare Workforce," *Quality and Safety in Healthcare* 12, no. 1 (2003): i2-i6. This legacy article is foundational to quality in healthcare. The article is available online at: https://qualitysafety.bmj.com/content/12/suppl_1/i2.

2. Write a report that describes five distinct historical and present-day factors that, according to Dr. Berwick, have inhibited improvements in healthcare. These factors should be stated in your own words and not copied verbatim from the article.

Tip: An example of one factor identified by Dr. Berwick is: Healthcare professionals and leaders are quick to blame individuals for performance gaps. In the article Dr. Berwick identifies many other inhibiting factors. Find five more different and distinct factors.

Defining a Performance Improvement Model

2

2.1 Plan a Rapid Cycle Improvement Project

Description

Rapid cycle improvement projects involve a series of Plan-Do-Study-Act (PDSA) improvement cycles to make incremental improvements in a process. Each improvement cycle involves a small process change and careful measurement of the effect of the change. In this case study you'll create a plan for an improvement cycle that can be completed in seven days.

Instructions

1. Conduct a seven-day improvement cycle for the following problem: Food in your refrigerator is often not eaten prior to the "Best Before" date and must be thrown out.

2. To start the cycle, write your answers to these three improvement questions:

   - What am I trying to accomplish? Be specific.
   - How will I know I have made an improvement? Provide a measurable definition of success.
   - What change can I make that will result in achieving what I want to accomplish? Be specific and identify the steps of a small process change that can be put in place and measured in just seven days.

Note: PDSA Directions and Examples can be found at: https://www.ahrq.gov/health-literacy /improve/precautions/tool2b.html

2.2   Measure the Effectiveness of an Improvement Project

Description

All improvement projects include a follow-up phase; that is, data are gathered to determine the effectiveness of action plans. In some instances, already existing performance measures can be used to evaluate results. In other situations, special studies of performance may be necessary. In this project you'll identify measures of performance for evaluating the effectiveness of an improvement project.

Background

Presume you are the quality manager in a hospital that conducted an improvement project to eliminate pulmonary complications in patients who develop dysphagia (difficulty swallow) following a stroke. The medical staff found that 45 percent of patients hospitalized following a cerebrovascular accident (stroke) had some degree of dysphagia and 10 percent of these patients developed pulmonary complications due to aspiration. A team of physicians, nurses, and physical therapists was convened to study the problem and implement changes for the purpose of eliminating all pulmonary complications for patients with dysphagia following a stroke. After studying how patients were being managed, the team agreed that improving the completeness and timeliness of nursing assessments and interventions would reduce pulmonary complications for patients who have strokes and secondary dysphagia.

To achieve the goal of zero pulmonary complications in patients with dysphagia following a stroke, the intensive care unit, medical ward nurses, and dieticians received in-service training in the following areas:

- How to conduct a complete and accurate assessment of patients to identify signs and symptoms of dysphagia.
- The importance of assessing stroke patients for gag reflex and swallowing on admission.
- The importance of promptly notifying the patient's attending physician within two hours if dysphagia signs or symptoms are identified.
- The importance of promptly notifying dietary services within two hours if dysphagia signs or symptoms are identified so the patient can be put on a special diet and a nutritional assessment conducted.

Instructions

1. Identify four process measures and one outcomes measure that could be used to evaluate the effectiveness of the actions taken to reduce pulmonary complications in the target population.

2.3   Performance Measurement Numerators and Denominators

Description

A performance measure is a "gauge used to assess the performance of a process or function of any organization" (CMS 2014). Most performance measures are a numerical rate, ratio, or proportion. To create these measures, two data elements are needed: a numerator and a denominator. A numerator is the upper portion of a fraction and a denominator is the lower portion of a fraction used to calculate a rate, proportion, or ratio. The numerator is a number that provides a magnitude (how much) and the denominator gives the number meaning (what). In this project you'll identify the numerator and denominator for measures of performance

Instructions

1. Download the answer sheet for this project from the AHMA student website.

2. For each of the behavioral healthcare performance measures listed below, describe the numerator and denominator that would be used to calculate the performance rate.

   - Percent of cases lacking a signed "Consent for Treatment" form.
   - Percent of inpatients for whom a follow-up appointment is scheduled within 2 weeks of discharge.
   - Percent of cases in which diagnostic criteria are based on the most recent edition of the *Diagnostic and Statistical Manual of Mental Disorders* (DSM).
   - Percent of clients with mental disorders that report acceptance/tolerance of their condition.
   - Percent of home care clients being seen for mental health services who maintain a Global Assessment of Functioning (GAF) score of less than 70.
   - Percent of clients six months following treatment for substance abuse that report addiction problems no longer interfere with their productive activities.
   - Average "order to report" time for diagnostic tests.

3. Record your responses on the answer sheet provided for this project.

Identifying Improvement Opportunities Based on Performance Measurement

3

3.1 Structure, Process, Outcome and Patient Experience Measures

Description

For a comprehensive understanding of performance, healthcare organizations measure four distinct characteristics: structure, process, outcome, and patient experience. Structure measures are used to assess the organization's capacity to provide quality patient care. Process measures are used to assess satisfactory completion of healthcare tasks. Outcome measures are used to assess the result of healthcare services. Patient experience measures are used to better understand how patients perceived the healthcare services. In this project you'll identify which characteristic (structure, process, outcome, or patient experience) is being evaluated by a performance measure.

Instructions

1. Download the answer sheet for this project from the AHIMA student website.
2. For each performance measure listed below, determine whether the measure is used to evaluate healthcare structure, process, outcome, or patient experience. The measures in this project are commonly used in ambulatory surgery centers.

   - Percentage of patients with a complete admission assessment (as defined by facility policy)
   - Percentage of patient records containing accurate insurance information
   - Percentage of surgeries that begin within 15 minutes of scheduled start time
   - Average length of stay from admission to discharge (in hours)
   - Percentage of patients requiring hospital admission following ambulatory surgery
   - Percent of patients whose systolic blood pressure varies more than 40mm Hg after admission to the post-anesthesia recovery unit

- Percentage of patients reportedly very satisfied with the ambulatory surgery admission process
- Number of surgeries cancelled due to unavailable equipment
- Percentage of patients who experience an adverse drug reaction
- Percentage of records containing documentation of preoperative evaluation by anesthesiologist
- Number of complaints received from patients/families about adequacy of parking accommodations
- Average charges for each of the top ten ambulatory procedures performed
- Percentage of patients that attend preoperative education classes
- Percentage of patients that develop a postoperative infection
- Number of health department citations for violations of health or safety regulations

3. Record your responses on the answer sheet provided for this project.

3.2   Measures of Process Performance

Description

Each step in the provision of health services can be measured to determine if performance is acceptable. In this project you'll identify measures of performance for steps in the hospital admissions process.

Instructions

1. Review the steps in the process of admitting a patient to the hospital for an elective procedure (shown in figure 3.1). The hospital admission process involves six distinct steps, five of which are under the control of the hospital admissions office. Satisfactory completion of steps 2 through 6 is important to the quality of patient care and patient satisfaction.

2. For each step, identify one process, outcome, or patient expectation measure that could be used by the manager of the hospital admissions office to evaluate how well employees are completing the step.

Figure 3.1: Process of admitting a patient to the hospital

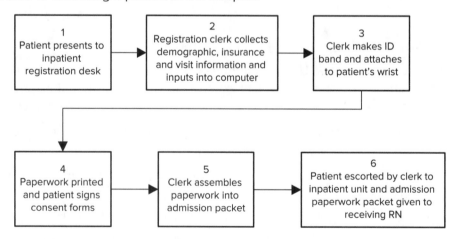

Using Teamwork in Performance Improvement 4

4.1 Managing Team Conflict

Description

It is critical to the success of an improvement project that the team leader has a strong understanding of best practices for avoiding team conflict and resolving conflict if it does happen.

Instructions

1. Read the following case study:
   When staff members were recruited for an improvement project, they were told the team's work would be additional to their regular work responsibilities but that they had to treat the project as a high priority. The members were expected to complete team assignments on time and were required to attend meetings. This was difficult because of other work responsibilities that also needed to be completed. Despite being aware of the expectations for the improvement project, by the third week of the project, team members started arriving late to meetings, making excuses for failing to complete their assigned tasks, and neglecting to return the team leader's phone calls.

2. If you were the team leader of the group described in case study, how would you refocus and motivate the team toward achieving the improvement goal? To answer this question, write a report that covers the following topics:

   - Your summary of the situation
   - Analysis of the cause of the poor performance
   - Actions you propose to take and why
   - Result you expect to see from your proposed actions
   - Method to measure the outcome of your actions.

Note: On the MindTools website (http://www.mindtools.com/pages/article/newTMM_79.htm) you'll find some fundamental principles of team conflict resolution. Use these principles along with other resources and teachings and your own professional experience to complete the report.

Aggregating and Analyzing Performance Improvement Data

5

5.1 Create a Cycle Time Data Collection Tool

Description

A key measure of process efficiency is cycle time, or the period required to complete a function, job, or task from start to finish. Cycle time is the result of systems and processes (how things are done). Thus, measures of cycle time are outcome measures. In this case study you'll create a data collection tool for gathering cycle time data.

Background

Presume you are the quality manager for a health system that includes an outpatient cystic fibrosis clinic. People with cystic fibrosis (CF) require frequent clinic visits to monitor their condition and receive support from a team of CF specialists.

Instructions

1. The clinic is conducting an improvement project to improve efficiency. Your task is to gather data. You must assist the project team collect information on patient flow in the clinic. The team wants to know what time a patient arrives at the clinic and what time they leave. In addition, they want to know how long it takes to complete activities that occur during their appointment. You ask the team for more specifics so you are sure the information gathered will meet their needs. The team states they want to know the average time between various steps in the clinic process. You determine the following data elements should be gathered on each patient during the study time period:

   - Time of the patient's scheduled appointment
   - Time patient leaves home to travel to the clinic

- Time patient arrives at the clinic
- Time patient checks in with receptionist
- Time patient is shown to the exam room
- Time nurse finishes clinical measurements (e.g., patient's weight, height, lung function)
- Time each CF team member comes into exam room to see patient and time they leave (CF team members include: physician, nurse, social worker, nutritionist, physical or respiratory therapy, and others)
- Time patient is ready to leave the clinic

2. You decide the best way to gather accurate information for the study is to ask receptionists and patients to record actual times on a data collection form. When a patient registers, the receptionist will ask what time the patient left home and what time they arrived at the clinic. The receptionist will record these times on the form along with the time of registration and the scheduled appointment date and time. The form will then be placed on a clipboard with a pencil attached and given to the patient with instructions to record the remaining times. The receptionist will explain why the data are needed and how to complete the form. If the patient does not have a watch, one will be provided. Before the patient leaves the clinic, they will be asked to return the clipboard and completed form (and watch, if one was provided) to the receptionist.

3. Design a data collection form that can be used to gather the data elements using the method described in step 2. The form should be easy to complete and self-explanatory.

5.2   Create and Interpret a Line Graph

Description

A line graph, sometimes called a run chart, is used to show changes in performance measurement data over several time periods. It can also be used for displaying several groups of continuous measurement data simultaneously. In this project you'll calculate performance measures, create a line graph of the measurement data, and interpret the results.

Instructions

1. Presume you are the quality director in a hospital. You've been asked to conduct a study for the nursing department. The purpose of the study is to determine how quickly nurses respond to patients' call lights (a device used by patients to communicate to nurses that assistance is needed). You gather from the hospital's automated Responder® 5 System which records all call data, including call-light usage and response times in seconds. The mean response time (in seconds) for each shift of the first 15 days of one month are shown in figure 5.1.

2. Using Excel™ or other graphic design software, create a line graph that shows the mean response time for each shift for each of the 15 days. Be sure to label the x- and y-axes in your graph and create a succinct title that describes the data being displayed.

3. Create a formal report of the study results for the director of nursing. Include the following information in the report:
- Purpose of the study
- How data were gathered (including sample size)
- Study results

- o the line graph you created in step 2 (insert the graph into your report)
- o a short narrative of the findings, including any significant performance patterns or trends that you may have been identified by analyzing the data

Figure 5.1: Daily mean response times

Shift	Daily Mean Responses Times (reported in seconds)														
	Day 1	Day 2	Day 3	Day 4	Day 5	Day 6	Day 7	Day 8	Day 9	Day 10	Day 11	Day 12	Day 13	Day 14	Day 15
Days	216	169	141	156	159	166	173	173	189	227	126	129	132	142	156
Evenings	122	121	178	183	138	115	144	119	153	149	155	124	147	168	132
Nights	85	96	86	103	101	119	92	99	89	112	92	82	102	101	113

5.3   Create a Histogram

Description

A histogram is used to show the frequencies of certain events or categories of data values in a set of data from one time period. Data are plotted in increasing or decreasing order based on the frequency count for each data categories. In this project you'll create a histogram from measurement data.

Instructions

1. Figure 5.2 is a data file containing the average number of minutes it took to code inpatient records each day in the health information management department. Data were collected for 30 days.
2. Calculate the range in coding times (highest to lowest) for the time period and the average number of minutes for the time period.
3. Use your calculations to create a histogram of the data.

Figure 5.2: Average time to code inpatient records (minutes)

DAY	TIME	DAY	TIME	DAY	TIME	DAY	TIME	DAY	TIME
1	30	7	31	13	27	19	31	25	33
2	31	8	29	14	31	20	30	26	30
3	30	9	28	15	28	21	28	27	31
4	27	10	34	16	30	22	26	28	29
5	32	11	29	17	32	23	28	29	32
6	33	12	30	18	29	24	30	30	31

5.4 Create a Pie Chart

Description

A pie chart shows a snapshot of performance from one time period. It graphically displays the relative frequency of variables in a data set. In this project you'll create a pie chart from measurement data.

Instructions

1. Figure 5.3 is a table showing the number of overtime hours paid to staff members working in departments that are part of the finance division of a hospital.

2. Create a pie chart from the data in the table. Label each slice and show the percentage of the whole pie each slice represents.

Figure 5.3: Staff overtime hours in the finance division for the last 12 months

Department	Number of overtime hours
Utilization review	742
Inpatient admissions	928
Business office	1103
Health information management	850
Outpatient admissions	519
Total Overtime Hours	**4142**

5.5 Create and Interpret a Bar Graph

Description

A bar graph is used to show performance measurement data from different time periods or different sites (for example, results from different facilities). In this project you'll create a bar graph from measurement data.

Instructions

1. Presume you are facilitating a Lean project team that is investigating ways to improve efficiency in the operating room (OR). The team discovered that surgeries do not always start at the scheduled time and this adversely affects staff productivity. To investigate why some surgeries do not start on time, the surgery department manager (a member of the Lean project team) asked five of her staff to collect data on the causes of delays. Data were gathered for six weeks and you receive the raw data. Now you need to create a report for the project team. First you summarize the data and create the table (figure 5.4).

2. Construct a bar graph from the data in the table. This will make it easier for the project team to quickly see the most common causes of delayed surgeries. The bar graph should illustrate the total number of delays in each cause category for the entire six-week period.

Figure 5.4: Causes of late starts for surgery cases

CAUSES	WK1	WK2	WK3	WK4	WK5	WK6
Transport-related delay	3	2	1	5	1	3
OR-related delay	4	3	3	4	5	4
Patient-related delay	3	2	5	5	2	7
Surgeon-related delay	2	3	2	3	2	1
Anesthesia-related delay	5	4	3	3	3	4
Other	2	2	1	1	2	1
TOTAL	19	16	15	21	15	20

3. Write a brief report for the Lean project team summarizing the findings.

Tip: To create the bar graph you'll need to calculate the total number of delays in each cause category.

5.6 Create and Interpret a Control Chart

Description

A control chart is special type of line graph that provides people with a statistical method for monitoring variation in performance measurement data. A control chart graphically depicts performance variations and helps people distinguish between common cause and special cause variation. In this project you'll create a control chart and interpret the results.

Instructions

Presume you are responsible for gathering performance measurement data in a 50-bed rural hospital. During the hospital's last state health department inspection, surveyors discover that more than 20 percent of patient records contained physician telephone orders that were not signed within 24 hours of receipt of the order (as required by state regulations). Your facility receives a citation for this problem.

Following the survey, unit clerks and nurses collaborate with physicians and their office staff to improve the timeliness of telephone order signatures. Three months after various strategies are put in place to eliminate the problem, you start collecting data to judge the effectiveness of these strategies. Each week, for 20 weeks, you review 20 patient records with telephone orders to determine how many of the charts have orders not signed within the required 24-hour time frame. Results of your data collection efforts are shown in figure 5.5.

To determine if the timeliness of telephone order signatures has improved and the process is stable you will create a p chart of the results to report to hospital administration. A p chart is used in statistical process control to track the proportion of a population (in this example, patient records with telephone orders is the population) that conforms or does not conform to requirements (in this case, untimely signatures).

Figure 5.5:   Records with late and unsigned physician orders

Week	Number of records reviewed	Number with late-signed/un-signed orders
1	20	1
2	20	1
3	20	0
4	20	2
5	20	1
6	20	0
7	20	0
8	20	3
9	20	2
10	20	1
11	20	1
12	20	0
13	20	1
14	20	5
15	20	1
16	20	0
17	20	3
18	20	2
19	20	2
20	20	1
Totals	400	27

1. Create a p chart showing the weekly results over the 20-week study period. Use the Excel template provided by your instructor to create the chart or create it without a template by completing the following steps:

   • Calculate the center line for the nonconformance rate for the study period. The center line is the average ($\bar{p}$) number of records that were found to be nonconforming for the entire study period (for example, did not meet signature timeliness requirements). Use the following formula to calculate the center line:

$$\bar{p} = \frac{\text{Total number of nonconforming records in samples being considered}}{\text{Total number of records reviewed in all samples being considered}}$$

- Calculate the 3 sigma upper control limit (UCL) and the lower control limit (LCL) for the nonconformance rates for the study period using the following formulas:

$$\text{UCL} \quad p = \bar{p} + 3\sqrt{\frac{\bar{p}(1-\bar{p})}{n}} \quad \text{LCL} \quad p = \bar{p} - 3\sqrt{\frac{\bar{p}(1-\bar{p})}{n}}$$

(Note: n is the number of items in each sample size)

- Create the control chart. It should contain each week's results, the center line, and the UCL and the LCL. Be sure to label the data increments on the y-axis, the week numbers on the x-axis, the center line, the UCL, and the LCL.

2. Create a report that answers the following questions:

- For the entire study period, what is the average number of noncompliant records?
- Compared to the earlier state survey findings, are phone orders now being signed more quickly by physicians?
- Is the process used to obtain telephone order signatures within 24 hours a stable process? For example, Did the average rate of nonconformance remain within the UCL and LCL during the 20-week study period?
- If the process is stable (in control), what could be done to further reduce the rate of nonconformance? If the process is unstable (out of control), what could be done to bring the process back into control (make it stable)?

5.7   Create and Interpret a Pareto Chart

Description

A Pareto chart is a specialized version of a histogram that ranks the categories from most frequent to least frequent. A Pareto chart provides an improvement team with information that helps them focus improvement efforts on the vital few problems rather than the trivial many. In this project you'll create a Pareto chart from measurement data and interpret the results.

Background

The data in the table (figure 5.6) were obtained from satisfaction surveys distributed to patients who had undergone a procedure in an ambulatory surgery center. The complaints are sorted into seven different categories (listed in the first column). In the second column is the number of times a patient complained about this aspect of their healthcare experience at the surgery center. Data were gathered over a 12-month time period.

Instructions

1. Create a Pareto chart from the data in the report. To create the chart, you'll need to calculate the percent of total and cumulative percent for each complaint category. Use the blank spaces on the form (figure 5.7) to record the numeric results of your calculations.

2. After creating the Pareto chart analyze the results and write a short narrative report identifying the complaints that need to be addressed first by the surgery center. Specifically, which complaints, if resolved, are likely to eliminate almost 78 percent of patient complaints about the surgery center?

Figure 5.6: Patient complaints about their ambulatory surgery experience

Complaint category	Frequency of response
Too noisy in unit	257
Inconvenient parking	190
Discharge instructions unclear	48
Admitting process too slow	38
Unable to schedule preop tests in evenings	296
Discharged too soon	86
All others	40
Grand total	**955**

Figure 5.7: Patient complaints about their ambulatory surgery experience

Complaint category	Frequency	Percent of total	Cumulative percent
Too noisy in unit	257		
Inconvenient parking	190		
Discharge instructions unclear	48		
Admitting process too slow	38		
Unable to schedule preop tests in evenings	296		
Discharged too soon	86		
All others	40		
Grand total	**955**	100	100

Communicating Performance Improvement Activities and Recommendations

6

6.1 Select Data Presentation Formats

Description

Measurement data can be displayed in many different graphic formats. When selecting a graph to use for reporting measurement data, several factors should be considered: the audience, intended use of the data, the basic message you want to communicate, and the underlying nature of the data and assumptions. Take these factors into consideration when completing this project. You'll be selecting the graph you would use to present measurement data for analysis purposes.

Instructions

1. Read the project case scenarios.

2. For each scenario identify an appropriate type of graph to use for reporting and analyzing the data discussed in the case.

Case 1: The hospital has collected patient satisfaction data for more than one year. It is now time for strategic planning and you've been asked to summarize the satisfaction data so that senior leaders can establish two or three strategic objectives related to improving patient satisfaction. They want to focus on the vital few issues that receive the lowest satisfaction ratings. What graph would you use to provide senior leaders with the information they need to establish strategic objectives related to patient satisfaction improvement?

Case 2: When a patient in the emergency department (ED) has an x-ray exam, the ED physician reviews the image and makes immediate treatment decisions. Within 12 hours, a radiologist is supposed to review the image and dictate a final report that is eventually filed with the patient's ED record. If the radiologist finds discrepancies and or findings that were overlooked by the ED physician, the ED is immediately notified. The physician director of the ED is concerned that radiologists are not reading x-ray films within 12 hours of an exam as required by hospital policy. He suspects that recent changes in the radiologists' schedule have caused an increase in the number of exams that are read beyond the 12-hour requirement. What graph would you use to show the director whether he is correct in his suspicions?

Case 3: You regularly collect data for the performance measure: Rate of vaginal birth after cesarean section (VBAC). This rate represents the proportion of women at the hospital who had a normal delivery after having a C-section for a prior birth. To create this rate, data are collected on the number of women having a VBAC and the total number of deliveries for women that had a previous C-section. Each month physicians in the OB-GYN department review the VBAC rate to determine if it varied significantly from last month's rate or the year-to-date average. They are particularly interested in any patterns or trends that might signal the need for more in-depth investigation. What graph would you use to support this monthly analysis?

Case 4: You have been asked by the medical director to investigate variations in patient wait times in the outpatient family practice clinic. The medical director wants to know if there is a correlation between the number of minutes patients must wait to see a physician and the time of the scheduled clinic appointment. Which graph tool would you use to help the medical director to determine if such a relationship exists?

Case 5: You've been asked to do a special study on physician compliance with pain management guidelines in the inpatient hospice unit. The medical staff executive committee has agreed that PRN (as needed) pain medication orders are not appropriate and has communicated this to all physicians. Your study will help the executive committee determine if physicians are complying with the medication ordering guidelines. You review ten patient records for each of the five physicians who admit patients to the hospice unit looking for pain medications ordered PRN. What graph would you use report the percent of noncompliant PRN pain medication orders written by each physician?

Project 6.2   Create a Corporate Report of Hospital Performance

Description

Members of a healthcare system commonly provide performance data to the corporate office for reporting to the health system board of trustees. In this project you'll create a board report using data submitted by providers in the health system.

Background

Presume you are the corporate quality and patient safety director for a 6-hospital health system. Each month the hospitals provide you with information about the number of "harmful" patient incidents that occurred the previous month. Harmful patient incidents can fall into one of five categories:

- Temporary harm, intervention required
- Temporary harm, initial or prolonged hospitalization
- Permanent patient harm
- Life sustaining intervention required
- Contributing to death

As you receive the data, it is entered into a spreadsheet. Throughout the year you create various summary and detailed reports for the corporate leaders.

Instructions

1. Download the data file for this project from the AHIMA student website.

2. The data file for this project contains 12 months of data from the six hospitals belonging to your health system. The file contains the monthly number of harmful patient incidents per 1,000 patient days for each hospital. Use this information to create *one* graph that provides the following information:

   - For each hospital, report the quarterly mean rate of harmful incidents (report the mean rate in each of the four quarters)
   - For the entire health system, report the quarterly mean rate of harmful incidents (report the mean rate in each of the four quarters)

   To create this graph, you'll first need to calculate the quarterly mean incident rate at each hospital. Then calculate the quarterly mean incident rate for the health system (all hospitals combined).

Tips: The purpose of the graph you are making is to show trends over time, including how the incident rates at each hospital varied throughout the year as well as how the incident rates for the whole health system varied throughout the year. Don't forget to label the graph with a title and other relevant information. The corporate leaders should be able to interpret the information in the graph without needing to refer to the raw data or read a narrative report.

Measuring Customer Satisfaction

7

7.1 Create a Survey Instrument

Description

A commonly used data collection tool is a survey or questionnaire. Surveys can be paper-based or electronic. In this project you'll develop a survey tool that will be used by the health information management (HIM) department in a large physician practice to judge customer satisfaction and identify improvement opportunities.

Background

You are the manager of the HIM department in a large physician clinic. The practice includes 35 primary care and specialty physicians and 9 nurse practitioners plus numerous medical office assistants and clerical staff. You want to measure how well the HIM department is meeting the needs of physicians and employees at the clinic. To do this, you want to develop a survey instrument that gathers answers to the following questions:

- Is the HIM department responding promptly to requests for information? If not, what types of requests are HIM employees slow to respond to?
- Are HIM department employees courteous in their interactions with physicians and people who work in the clinic? If not, what opportunities for improvement exist?

You know that people are busy and won't complete a long survey. Therefore, you'll want to gather as much information as possible using a short (one page or less) survey instrument.

Instructions

1. Create a survey instrument to gather information for this performance measurement project.

7.2 Query an Online Data Source of Patient Experience Measure Results

Description

In this project you'll learn how to query an online database of patient experience measures and report the results.

Background

Presume you work in the quality management department at a nearby hospital. You know the results of patient satisfaction surveys are publicly available on the Internet and consumers in your market area can get this data. You want the hospital leaders and the governing board to see what the data reveal about the hospital where you work and how it compares to other hospitals in the state and to hospitals throughout the U.S. You'll use data on the *Why Not the Best* website to create a report for hospital leaders.

   The report you will create includes the measures of "the Hospital Consumer Assessment of Healthcare Providers and Systems (HCAHPS). This survey asks a random sample of recently discharged patients about important aspects of their hospital experience" (CMS 2021).

Instructions

1. Go to the Commonwealth website, *Why Not the Best* (http://whynotthebest.org).

2. Use the search function on this site to retrieve the data you need to create a report. Choose a nearby hospital (or the hospital that has been assigned by your instructor). Find the most recent data for the measures in the category entitled, "Patient Experience (HCAHPS)." You will need the data for the hospital, the state where the hospital is located, and the entire U.S. There are several measurement results to determine:

   - Percent of patients that were highly satisfied
   - Percent who reported that doctors always communicated well
   - Percent who reported that nurses always communicated well
   - Percent who reported they always received help as soon as they wanted
   - Percent who reported that staff always explained about medicines
   - Percent who reported that pain was always well controlled
   - Percent who reported that their room was always kept quiet at night
   - Percent who reported that their room and bathroom was always kept clean
   - Percent who reported that they were given information about recovery at home
   - Percent who reported that they would definitely recommend this hospital to friends and family (CMS 2023).

3. Create a data table for hospital leadership that shows the results for each question for the hospital, the state and the nation. Format the table so it is easy for the leaders to compare the hospital's results with state and national results. Include the time period in which the data were reported.

Note: You can access the data to complete the report without signing up for an account on the site. If you do sign-up (it's free) you'll be able to download the data. Otherwise, you'll only be able to view the search results. The search function on this site is self-explanatory, however if you need assistance use the "help" function on the site.

7.3   Measure Customer Satisfaction with an Important HIM Process

Description

To evaluate the quality of services provided by the HIM department, the manager will want to know if important activities are meeting customers' needs. In this project you'll review a HIM department process, identify customers of the process and their needs, and select process measures that can be used by the manager to evaluate whether customer needs are being met.

Instructions

1. Review the steps in the process of importing a paper document from another source into the electronic health record (EHR) of a clinic patient (figure 7.1). This is an important HIM department process because timely provider access to patient information from all sources is a vital component of quality patient care.

2. Answer the following questions:

   - Who are the customers of the clinic HIM department process illustrated in this flowchart?

   - What is important to the customers of this process? For example, what are their needs and expectations?

   - What activities in the process must be performed well in order to meet the needs and expectations of process customers?

   - What are three measures of performance that can be used to determine whether this process is meeting customers' needs and expectations? What is the numerator and denominator for each measure?

Figure 7.1: Flowchart of x-ray process

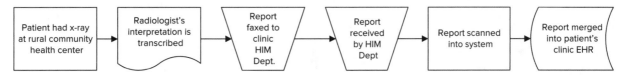

Refining the Continuum of Care

8.1 Analyze Hospital Efficiency Profile

Description

Data illustrating resource use among healthcare organizations can be presented in many different formats. The most common are tables and graphs. In this project you'll learn about a graphic format commonly used to present utilization comparison data and you'll interpret the information on the graph.

Instructions

1. The diagram (figure 8.1) illustrates comparisons among seven hospitals for length of stay and charges for patients with a final diagnosis of viral meningitis without cc/mcc (DRG 076). This report is used to evaluate the efficiency of seven different hospitals with your hospital being compared to the others. Where your hospital and the other hospitals fall on the efficiency chart is indicated with a dot.

2. Using information provided in the diagram, write a report that includes the following information:

   - Hospital with the longest length of stay
   - Hospital with the shortest length of stay
   - Hospital with the highest charges
   - Hospital with the lowest charges
   - Hospital that is most inefficient, provide the rationale for your answer
   - Hospital that is most efficient, provide the rationale for your answer

Figure 8.1: Hospital efficiency report

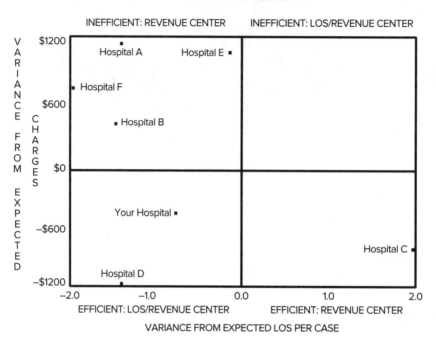

Project 8.2 Identify Medical Appropriateness Guidelines

Description

Criteria used for utilization management purposes are often derived from nationally published practice guidelines/recommendations. In this project you'll locate treatment recommendations relevant to a particular patient population and interpret the recommendations.

Background

Presume you are the quality manager in a general surgery outpatient clinic. The business office manager comes to you with a reimbursement problem. A health plan has denied payment for three claims involving drainage of non-painful fluid-filled breast cysts in female patients. All are patients of a surgeon who recently moved from another state and joined the clinic nine months ago. The other clinic physicians do not routinely drain non-painful breast cysts that are confirmed by ultrasound as harmless fluid filled sacs. The new physician says that in her experience drainage of these cysts help relieve patients' anxiety and fear the lesion could become cancerous. The business office manager doesn't know how the surgeon should respond to the payment denials and asks you to research appropriate treatment options for patients with non-painful fluid-filled breast cysts.

Instructions

1. Locate the most recently published practice guideline for treatment of patients with non-painful fluid-filled breast cysts. Guidelines can be found by searching on the phrase, "non-painful fluid-filled breast cysts."

2. Obtain a complete copy of the most recent guidelines. Write a memo to the business office manager to share with the surgeon that includes the following information:

- Group that published the guideline
- Year the guideline was published
- Where the guideline can be found online (site name and URL)
- Based on the guideline recommendations:
  - Is drainage an appropriate treatment for patients with a non-painful fluid-filled breast cyst?
  - Are there any circumstances that might make this treatment appropriate?
  - Should the surgeon challenge the insurance payment denials or not? If yes, how should the challenge be worded? If no, how should the surgeon change her practices going forward? Is there something she can do differently to comply with the guidelines?

8.3   Use Criteria to Evaluate Appropriate Use of Healthcare Services

Description

Providers and health plans use decision support tools – utilization guidelines – to assist in making decisions about the most appropriate care for specific conditions and diagnoses, as well as prevent overuse and guard against underuse. In this project you'll apply utilization guidelines to evaluate the appropriateness of healthcare services.

Background

Presume you are a health plan utilization review coordinator. Your responsibilities involve evaluating the medical necessary of services, including admissions to rehabilitation facilities. The utilization guidelines to evaluate appropriateness of patient admissions for orthopedic rehabilitative care following a hospital stay for a fractured hip, total knee or total hip replacement include several key points:

- Patient is medically stable at time of transfer:
  - Patient is free of fever, and
  - Patient is not ventilator dependent.
and
- Patient demonstrates rehabilitation potential:
  - Capable of participation in a minimum of 3 hours of therapy per day (physical and occupational therapies combined), and
  - Potential for learning and carryover demonstrated in acute care, and
  - Requires therapy from two or more disciplines, and
  - Requires intensity of services not available from home health or an outpatient facility.

Before approving insurance coverage for post-hospital admission to a rehabilitation facility for orthopedic rehabilitation, all the above criteria must be met. If one or more criteria are not met, you will send the request to the health plan medical director who will make the final decision as to whether the rehabilitative care will have prior approval for payment by the health plan. The patient and attending physician can appeal payment denials by providing additional information.

Instructions

1. Download the answer sheet for this project from the AHIMA Student website.

2. Review the five case scenarios provided. Presume you have been contacted by the hospital case manager in the case scenario to request insurance authorization for the patient to be transferred to a rehabilitation facility. How would you respond to this request? Use the above criteria to judge whether orthopedic rehabilitation would be medically appropriate for the patient described in the case.

3. If the patient does not meet one or more admission appropriateness criteria, which criteria are not met? Use the answer sheet provided for the project to document your responses.

Case 1: A 72-year-old bed-ridden female with Alzheimer's disease and other comorbid conditions was admitted to the hospital following a fall at the foster care home where she lives. She suffered a non-displaced fracture of her left hip. Due to the patient's advanced coronary artery disease and other comorbid conditions, it was determined by her physician that surgical intervention would not be appropriate. She was kept in traction for six days while her cardiac condition was closely monitored. During the hospitalization, she received physical therapy twice a day to increase her upper extremity strength although she was not able to fully participate in therapy. On day seven of her hospitalization the patient is ready for discharge and the case manager calls you to request prior authorization of insurance benefits for post-hospital orthopedic rehabilitation.

Case 2: A 82-year-old female was admitted for an elective left knee replacement. The patient lives independently in an apartment in an assisted living retirement center although she has a history of difficulties ambulating due to degenerative arthritis in both knees. No one lives in the apartment with her. Her past medical history includes mitral valve replacement at age 76 and laparoscopic cholecystectomy at age 70. She is on multiple medications, including Coumadin, which was stopped seven days prior to surgery. She underwent surgery on the day of admission. Her postoperative course was uneventful except for hard-to-control postoperative pain. Physical therapy started on day two of her hospital stay and occupational therapy started on day three. She was able to participate fully in all therapies. Her ambulation and ability to care for herself slowly improved. The patient is ready for hospital discharge on the seventh postoperative day and the case manager calls you to request prior authorization of insurance benefits for post-hospital orthopedic rehabilitation.

Case 3: A 62-year-old man was admitted to the hospital for an elective hip replacement. He has a history of alcoholism, chronic obstructive pulmonary disease (COPD), and degenerate joint disease. Prior to admission, he lived independently with his wife of 32 years. The patient underwent surgery on the day of admission. His postoperative course was complicated by pulmonary congestion requiring respiratory therapy treatments. Despite this complication, he was able to begin physical and occupational therapy 24 hours postoperatively. On the fourth hospital day, the patient developed a COPD exacerbation and pneumonia for which he was given Prednisone and IV antibiotics. This complication caused him to miss three physical therapy treatments. By the ninth postoperative day, the patient was afebrile and able to ambulate ten feet with assistance and perform some routine self-care activities. His physician orders discharge on the ninth postoperative day with plans for continued physical therapy post-discharge. His physician documents that patient can fully participate in the therapy. The case manager calls you to request prior authorization of insurance benefits for post-hospital orthopedic rehabilitation.

Case 4: A 37-year-old man was admitted to the hospital for an elective right knee replacement. He had undergone replacement of his left knee six months earlier. Knee replacements were needed because of the patient's severe degenerative arthritis. The patient has a history of smoking and recurrent bronchitis, but no other comorbid conditions. He lives with his 62-year-old mother. The patient underwent surgery on the day of admission. Physical therapy was begun 24 hours postoperatively. By day five, the patient was able to ambulate independently twenty feet using crutches. His physician ordered continued physical therapy post-discharge. The patient is ready for discharge on the third day of his hospital stay and the case manager calls you to request prior authorization of insurance benefits for post-hospital orthopedic rehabilitation.

Case 5: A 51-year-old female was admitted to the hospital for an elective right knee replacement for degenerative joint disease. The patient has a history of Type I diabetes and obesity. She lives with her 55-year-old husband who can care for her. She was admitted the night before surgery. Her surgery was uneventful and physical therapy was begun 24 hours postoperatively. On day three of her hospitalization, she spiked a fever to 101.2 degrees Fahrenheit and was found to have pulmonary atelectasis. Respiratory therapy treatments and IV antibiotics were started. Due to her decreased endurance, she was only able to tolerate brief periods of assisted ambulation. Her physician ordered a nutritional consultation and diabetic teaching. Six days following her surgery, her strength began to return and by the ninth day, she was able to participate in physical therapy three times a day for 45 minutes and occupational therapy once a day to improve her self-care skills. Her diabetes was under control. On the 11th hospital day, her physician feels the patient is ready for discharge with plans for continued rehabilitative services. The case manager calls you to request prior authorization of insurance benefits for post-hospital orthopedic rehabilitation.

Improving the Provision of Care, Treatment, and Services

9

9.1 Performance Measures for a Home Health Agency

Description

In this project you'll identify performance measures for a home health agency.

Background

Imagine you have been hired as quality manager for a soon-to-open home health agency. The business manager asks you to select performance measures that can be used to judge the quality of care that will be provided to home health patients. You go to the Centers for Medicare and Medicaid Services (CMS) Measures Inventory Tool website to find measures that would be relevant for use in a home health agency. So agency management won't be overwhelmed at the start with too many measures, you decide to select two process measures, two outcome measures, and one patient reported outcome measure.

Instructions

1. Download the answer sheet for this project from the AHIMA student website.
2. Go to the CMS Measures Inventory Tool website (https://cmit.cms.gov/CMIT_public/ListMeasures). Use the search function to find measures of performance for a home health agency and measures in each of the categories. Only measures found using this search function in the CMS Measures Inventory should be used to complete the assignment.
3. In the first column of the answer sheet provided below list the measures you found on the CMS website. The measure title is at the top of the page describing each measure. Be sure you write the measures in descriptive "measurement" terms. The measure should start with words or phrases such as: "percent of," "number of," "mean rate," and the like.

4. Identify the numerator and denominator that are used to create each measure. Read though the description of the measure on the website and you'll find this information. Figure 9.1 is an example of how one row on the answer sheet would be completed for a process measure from the CMS Measure Inventory that could be used in an inpatient rehabilitation facility.

Figure 9.1: Measure numerator and denominator

Measure	Numerator	Denominator
Process: *Percent of patients/residents with an admission and a discharge functional assessment and a care plan that addresses function.*	*Number of patient/resident stays with functional assessment data for each self-care and mobility activity and at least one self-care or mobility goal.*	*Number of Medicare Part A covered resident stays*

9.2   Identify Measurement Data for Outcomes Management Initiative

Description

The Plan-Do-Study-Act (PDSA) performance improvement model is often used for an outcomes management initiative. During the "Study" phase of the model, data are gathered to determine whether actions taken to improvement performance (the "Do" phase) have been successful. In this project you'll determine how to gather information to check the effectiveness of improvement actions.

Background

Presume you are the director of health information management in a 250-bed urban hospital. To improve the health of elderly people living in the community, the hospital undertakes an outcomes management project intended to improve the rate of pneumococcal and influenza vaccinations for individuals age 65 and older. From August through October, the hospital sponsors a community awareness campaign to encourage greater use of pneumococcal and influenza vaccinations among people 65 years and older. This campaign includes articles in the local newspaper and health fairs to inform the general public. An educational session for primary care physicians is held to provide information about immunizing elderly patients. In May of the following year the geriatric case manager comes to you for information as to whether the outcomes management project was successful. Specifically, did the number of patients hospitalized for immunization-preventable pneumonia and influenza during the winter months decrease from the previous year's numbers? Data are to be gathered only on patients 65 years and older.

Instructions

1. Write a report that includes the following information:

   - Characteristics of patients that would be included and excluded from your data collection efforts
   - *International Classification of Diseases, Tenth Revision, Clinical Modification* (ICD-10-CM) codes that would be used to identify patients admitted to the hospital for treatment of immunization-preventable pneumonia and influenza
   - Source of data to be used to determine the number of hospital admissions for immunization-preventable pneumonia and influenza during the winter months.

Preventing and Controlling Infectious Disease

10

10.1 Create and Analyze a Process Flowchart

Description

A flowchart is a graphic representation of how a process works. For performance improvement purposes, a flowchart helps people clarify how things are currently working and how they could be improved. In this project you'll create a flowchart for a work process and identify opportunities for improving the efficiency of the process.

Instructions

1. Read the description of the hospital cancer registry process for case finding, abstracting, and reporting cancer cases (see "Process Description").

2. Create a detailed flowchart of the process, as described. The flowchart should include at least the following symbols:

   Start / End   ( )   Decision   ◇ No / Yes

   Process Step   [ ]

   Other flowchart symbols may be used as appropriate.

3. When the flowchart is complete, review the steps in the process and write a report that answers the following questions:

   • Are there bottlenecks in the process? At which step(s)?

   • Are there redundant steps that can be combined? Which ones?

- Is there idle time in the process? At which step(s)?
- Is there backtracking in the workflow? At which step(s)?
- Does the process include re-work that can be eliminated? At which step(s)?

Process Description

Step 1: Case Finding. Case finding is the process of finding new cancer cases diagnosed within a given time period; it is the first step in the cancer reporting system. It applies to all patients—inpatients and outpatients—if they are diagnosed and/or treated with a reportable tumor. Registrars use several data sources for case findings. Most cases (90–95 percent) are identified through pathology reports. Pathology reports are useful because they contain detailed information about the cancer (such as diagnosis, histology, and behavior). Some facilities use additional sources for case finding, such as hospital admission and discharge records, surgery schedules, cytology reports, oncology reports (nuclear and medical), radiology reports, and financial billing records. These sources, however, are less informative than pathology reports, and registrars often use multiple sources or refer to patient health records to find the information they need. All sources are reviewed, however, to ensure a report does not contradict findings from another report.

Only new cases of cancer are added to the registry. Information about patients with the same type of cancer who are already in the registry is follow-up information and a new case abstract is not initiated.

Step 2: Add to Suspense File. Once a case is confirmed as reportable and a new case, it is added to a suspense file to await abstraction. In most facilities, case finding is performed weekly or monthly, but cases may reside in the suspense file for up to six months before abstraction. The rationale for this is to wait for tests and treatments to be performed and added to the EHR.

The first case entered into the suspense file will be the first case abstracted. However, procedures and treatments can be done at different speeds, depending on factors such as the cancer type, cancer stage, and facility resources. Using a standard waiting time for all cases creates an unnecessary delay if treatments are made available earlier than prior cases. Adding a notification system to inform registrars of when treatments are available will enable them to abstract the case as soon as the treatment is available, instead of using a fixed period for all cases.

Figure 10.1:   Estimated time for step 1 and 2

Activity time		Non-activity/wait time	
Step	Time	Step	Time
Step 1: Case finding from pathology reports	Daily: 1 hour	Step 2: Suspense File	3–6 months. Varies among hospitals
Step 1: Case finding from ICD-10 list and other sources	Monthly: 1 day	Step 2: Suspense File	An average of 15 days for hospitals with 300 or more reportable cases a year.

Step 3: Abstract the Case. While case finding generally provides an overview of the case, itself, abstracting is more comprehensive and detailed. Abstracting uses different parts of patient health records to collect demographic information, tumor-related information, and information about staging, diagnostic studies, and treatment. Much of the same data reviewed during the case finding process is analyzed again during the abstraction process.

The patient's data is not always available in local health records. This happens when patients receive care at different hospitals/facilities. Abstraction of cases requiring data retrieval from external sources takes longer to complete. It may be difficult to access information from facilities outside the organization's network. When electronic access is not available, phone calls may be used to contact outside facilities and this can be problematic if nurses and physicians are unwilling to share patient information due to their concerns about privacy. After all the required information is collected and the abstract is considered complete, it is saved in the suspense file in preparation for submission to the central state registry.

Step 4: Submit to Central Registry. Completed abstracts are sent to the state registry at fixed intervals. Facilities with a higher number of cases are required to report to the state registry at a higher frequency. For example, facilities with an annual caseload of 300 or more may be required to report monthly, while facilities with an annual caseload of 150–299 may be required to report every other month. Source: Jabour, Abdulrahman M., Brian E. Dixon, Josette F. Jones, David A. Haggstrom. 2018. "Toward Timely Data for Cancer Research: Assessment and Reengineering of the Cancer Reporting Process." *JMIR Cancer*, 4, no. 1. doi: 10.2196/cancer.7515.

Decreasing Risk Exposure

11

11.1 Create a Cause-and-Effect Diagram for an Improvement Project

Description

A cause-and-effect diagram is a structured brainstorming tool used to generate and sort ideas or hypotheses about possible causes of problems. Items are listed in a graphic display sometimes called a fishbone diagram (because of its shape). In this project you'll create a cause-and-effect diagram to use during an improvement project.

Background

Presume you are the quality director at a hospital. In surveys of satisfaction patients are often unhappy with the food. Patient complaints about receiving cold food were 35 percent of the total negative comments in last quarter's survey results. Administration decides to take action to solve this problem. A team of the people involved in the food delivery process (nursing staff and dietary aides) is formed and you are asked to lead the improvement project. The team meets to discuss the problem of cold food being delivered to patients. They start the project by constructing a high-level flowchart of the hospital's food ordering and delivery process (figure 11.1).

Next, the team develops a cause-and-effect diagram to identify all possible causes of the undesirable effect (cold food). Causes are brainstormed and sorted into major cause categories on the diagram.

Instructions

1. Obtain a cause-and-effect diagram template. Your instructor may provide you with a template or you can download one from the Internet. Here are two sites where free templates can be found:
   http://templatelab.com/fishbone-diagram-templates/
   https://www.template.net/business/word-templates/fishbone-diagram-template/

Figure 11.1:   High level flow chart of food ordering and delivery

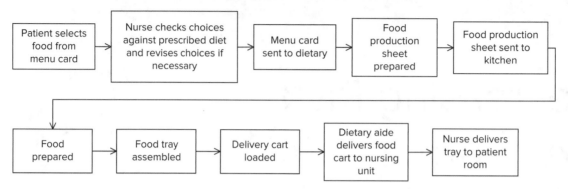

2. Using your cause-and-effect diagram template, brainstorm all possible reasons why you think food might be cold when it is delivered to a hospitalized patient. It's okay to be creative. This is *your* opinion as to what might be causing delivery of cold food.

3. Record the causes in the appropriate category on the diagram (people, methods, materials, or environment).

4. Write a brief report describing the next step the team should take after completing the cause-and-effect diagram.

11.2   Evaluate Publicly Available Patient Safety Measurement Data

Description

Data for several measures of patient safety are publicly available. Whether consumers find these data useful for making provider choices is unclear. In this project you'll review measures on a consumer-oriented patient safety website.

Instructions

1. Explore the most current list of hospital performance measures of patient safety found on the website of the Leapfrog Group (http://www.leapfroggroup.org).

2. Write a report covering the following topics:

- What aspect(s) of safety (structure, process, outcome, patient experience) are being evaluated by the Leapfrog patient safety measures? List the measures found on the site and the aspect of safety being measured.

- What "value" do these publicly reported measures add to an individual hospital's existing information about patient safety? Explain your answer.

- As a consumer of healthcare services, are you more interested in knowing a hospital's rate of adverse events/medical errors or ratings on the Leapfrog patient safety measures? Explain your answer.

11.3 Classify Patient Incidents

Description

Patient incident report forms completed by staff in a healthcare organization are a primary source of information on patient safety. Information gleaned from these reports is regularly summarized and communicated to clinical and administrative leaders by the quality or risk management department. In this project you'll categorize patient incidents for reporting purposes.

Background

Presume you are a data analyst in a hospital quality department. One of your job responsibilities is to review patient incident reports as they are received in the department to gather information for a monthly report to administration. This report includes the number of incidents that occurred in each of the following three categories:

- Level 1 event: an incident that resulted in patient death or serious short- or long-term (6 weeks or more) disability or harm
- Level 2 event: an incident that resulted in minimal short-term patient disability or harm
- Level 3 event (near miss): an incident that could have resulted in patient death, disability or harm but did not, either by chance or through timely intervention

Instructions

1. Read the ten patient incident descriptions that accompany this project. For each incident, indicate how it should be categorized (according to the definitions provided). If the description contains insufficient information to allow it to be categorized, indicate that "more information is needed." If you are not familiar with the terminology used in the incident descriptions consult a medical dictionary.

Incident Descriptions

Incident 1

The nursing staff was providing a patient with routine morning care. This consisted of showering the patient in the shower room on the ward. The patient was being washed while seated in a chair when he slid off the chair hitting his face, hip, and shoulder. The patient was examined by the doctor at 7:55 a.m. and transferred to the emergency department (ED) for further evaluation. The ED physician ordered x-rays. No fractures were found however he did have some minor contusions. The patient was returned to the ward where neurological checks were initiated per policy and reported as normal.

Incident 2

A 61-year-old female was admitted for gastrointestinal bleeding and underwent hemicolectomy. She was put on a ventilator postoperatively and transferred to the surgical intensive care unit. On the eighth post-operative day, while still on the ventilator, the patient developed copious respiratory secretions and became restless and agitated. She was sedated with Diprivan which seemed to improve her condition. On the ninth post-operative day two nurses turned the patient on her side for a bath. The patient started coughing and was noted to have copious secretions. A respiratory therapist was summoned to assist the nurses who had already started to suction the patient's secretions. The respiratory therapist checked the patient's endotracheal tube and found it to be in the oropharynx rather than the trachea. The tube was removed, and the respiratory therapist attempted re-intubation but was not successful. A "code red" (cardiac arrest) was called to alert professional staff that help was needed. A certified nurse anesthetist arrived within minutes and attempted to reintubate the patient, but he could not visualize the patient's vocal cords (patient had very large tongue). Another attempt was made with a smaller tube, and this was also unsuccessful. The third reintubation attempt was successful; however, the patient could not be resuscitated, and she expired.

Incident 3

Level 3

The following incident was reported in the Journal of Anesthesiology, by which a "two-year-old boy with retroperitoneal rhabdomyosarcoma was scheduled to undergo abdominal MRI. Anesthesia was provided by an anesthesiologist/nurse team with experience in anesthesia for MRI. After a check for removal of all ferromagnetic materials and of the MRI compatible ventilator, anesthesia was induced and maintained via a closely fitting facemask in the spontaneously breathing child using sevoflurane-nitrous oxide in 50% oxygen, and vital signs were monitored using MRI-safe equipment (graphite electrocardiogram leads, fiberoptic pulse oximetry, end-expiratory carbon dioxide, noninvasive blood pressure). When a low level of sevoflurane was noted in the vaporizer, the nurse was asked to refill it. However, because a refill bottle of sevoflurane was not immediately found, the nurse instead carried a portable sevoflurane vaporizer from the induction room into the MRI suite. Neither she nor the anesthesiologist considered that the almost empty sevoflurane vaporizer in the MRI suite was fixed to the ventilator and hence could not be replaced at all. When the nurse put the vaporizer on the examination table, it was rapidly attracted toward the MRI's 1.5-T magnet. It was only by the force of four hands that the vaporizer could be directed to strike against the gantry instead of flying directly into the magnet, where it might have hit the child. The table with the sleeping child was rapidly moved out of the gantry, avoiding further danger. Neither the child nor the MRI machine was harmed, and the examination went on without further complications after excluding MRI damage and refilling the fixed vaporizer." (Zimmer et al. 2004)

Incident 4

Need more info

A 59-year-old patient with chronic obstructive pulmonary disease was ordered by his physician to have 100% oxygen via facemask to correct his low PaO2. The patient's condition did not improve despite being on the 100% oxygen for one hour. When the physician entered the patient's room and moved the bed to begin intubation, it was discovered the patient was not on oxygen. Rather the oxygen tubing was attached to the medical air flow meter. Once the oxygen tube was connected to the oxygen flow meter the patient's condition improved. No further action was required.

Incident 5

Level 2

A 35-year-old patient with left shoulder pain was seen in the physical therapy department for treatment of left shoulder and neck pain. His physician had prescribed several therapy modalities: hot packs, phonophoresis with ultrasound 1.5 watts per square centimeter and hydrocortisone 1% for 8 minutes, massage, and interferential electrical stimulation. When the patient arrived for his first treatment, there were four other patients in the department at the time. He received electrical stimulation and hot packs to his left shoulder, followed by ultrasound. Following the patient's therapy, the staff noted a reddened area on his left shoulder. The patient had been advised to report excessive heat from the treatment, but he said he hadn't felt anything too hot. No treatment for the redness was deemed necessary and it was gone five days later when the patient came in for a second appointment.

Incident 6

Level 3

Two weeks after being admitted to the hospital's Alzheimer Unit, a 67-year-old patient wandered away from the facility. He was last seen at approximately 4:30 p.m. and was not in his room when dinner was delivered. The patient's nurse first looked for him in the outside hallways and other patient rooms. When he could not be located, the nurse contacted security. A full search of the building and grounds was initiated and lasted about an hour. When the patient was not found, the local police department was notified of his missing status along with a physical description and information about his condition. The next morning the city police discovered the man wandering downtown (about four miles from the hospital). He was taken to the emergency department for evaluation where he was found to be dehydrated and suffering from pneumonia. He was admitted to the hospital for treatment and later transferred back to the Alzheimer Unit after six days of hospitalization.

Incident 7

Level 3

A laparotomy sponge was left in a patient who had undergone an esophagogastrectomy and thoracotomy. At the end of the esophagogastrectomy, sponge counts done by the surgical nurse were reported as correct and the surgeon proceeded with the thoracotomy. At the end of the thoracotomy, the surgical nurse discovered the sponge count was incorrect by one sponge. A portable chest x-rays was done and erroneously read as negative by the surgeon (no radiologist was available in-house to interpret the x-ray). The next day the x-ray was read by a radiologist who found that a foreign object had been left in the patient's chest. The patient was returned to the operating room for removal of the sponge. According to the surgeon, this second procedure prolonged the patient's hospital stay by three days.

Incident 8

Needs more info

A nine-year-old girl was admitted to the pediatric unit with acute lymphocytic leukemia. This was a new diagnosis for this patient. Following six weeks of chemotherapy in the hospital, her immune system became extremely compromised. She was maintained in an isolation room for the last three weeks of therapy as her white count had dropped to very low levels. During week six in the hospital, the child spiked a fever to 104°F and became tachycardic. She complained of a new onset of pain in her head. This was reported to the oncologist immediately and cultures were obtained from blood, nasopharynx (NP), and spinal fluid. The spinal fluid and NP cultures grew Aspergillus fumigatus. Despite aggressive treatment, the child was taken to the operating room for removal of her left eye and cheekbone to prevent further damage from the Aspergillus. She was ultimately discharged home.

Incident 9

Level 2

A nurse on the medical ward tried to start an IV on a 72-year-old patient but was unsuccessful because the patient became agitated and moved around constantly. This occurred toward the end of the nurse's shift, and she notified the incoming nurse that she had been unable to start the IV. The incoming nurse said she would try to do it as soon as she finished passing out medications to her other assigned patients. When the incoming nurse finally got around to entering the room of the patient who needed to have the IV started, she discovered that the first nurse had not removed the tourniquet from the patient's arm. This was four hours after the original nurse had tried but failed to begin the IV. The patient's arm was swollen and there was some residual neurological and vascular damage that was still present at the time the patient was discharged.

Incident 10

Level 3

A female patient was scheduled for a phacoemulsification, cataract extraction, and an intraocular lens implantation on her right eye. Just prior to her operation, the anesthesiologist administered a lid block and partial retrobulbar injection to the patient's left eye even though her right eye was the operative site. The mistake was discovered by the surgeon before making an incision. The patient's right eye was anesthetized and surgically prepared and the surgery proceeded without incident.

11.4   Report Patient Safety Measurement Data

Description

An important quality management skill is knowing how to turn raw data into a performance report that is useful for decision-makers. In this project you'll be doing just that.

Instructions

1. Download the data file for this project from the AHIMA student website.

2. The data file is an Excel™ spreadsheet containing information about all reported patient incidents in a hospital for a one-month period in July. Each incident is listed on a separate row. Using the information in the data file, you'll create two reports. One is for the hospital's vice president of nursing and one is for the board of trustees. Below is a description of the information to be included in each report and the format to be used to display the information.

   Incident Report .for the VP of nursing: This report includes only patient incident information from those units where nurses care for patients (Medical Inpatient, Surgery Inpatient, Pediatric Inpatient, Psych Inpatient, Intensive Care Unit, Coronary Care Unit, Emergency Services, Operating Room, Post Anesthesia Recovery Unit and Surgical Outpatient). For *each* unit, report:

   - total number of incidents in each event category
   - percent of incidents in each event category
   - total number of incidents in each severity category
   - percent of incidents in each severity category

   The report for the VP of nursing should be a numeric report using a tabular format (sometimes called a data table). It is not an aggregate summary of incidents in all nursing units. The data are to be reported for each unit.

   Incident report for the board of trustees: This report includes patient incident information from *all* units in the hospital. The board report should include:

   - total number of incidents in each event category
   - percent of incidents in each event category
   - total number of incidents in each severity category
   - percent of incidents in each severity category

   The report for the Board should be a graphic data display (for example, bar graph, line graph, and the like).

3. Include titles, time frames, and other informative information in the reports.

Tips: You'll want to create reports that communicate all the information required (per instructions). Generally, students create anywhere from 1-4 tabular numeric reports for the VP of nursing and 1-4 graphs for the board of trustees' report. The ideal would be only one tabular report for the VP of nursing and only one graph for the board of trustees.

11.5   Conduct a Root Cause Analysis of a Sentinel Event

Description

A root cause analysis (RCA) is a structured improvement project that involves investigation of a significant adverse patient incident or sentinel event. The goal of an RCA is to identify and fix the underlying causes of the event. In this project you'll review the circumstances surrounding a sentinel event, identify the root causes, and select actions for preventing similar events in the future.

Instructions

1. Read the sentinel event summary provided with this project. The summary describes circumstances surrounding a wrong procedure event. This incident happened at a hospital in the Midwest.

2. Research the literature and conduct an Internet search to identify the common causes of wrong procedure errors such as the one described in this incident.

3. Research the literature and conduct an Internet search to identify process changes that are recommended for preventing the type of error that is described in this incident.

4. Write a report that includes the following information:

   - Departments or disciplines that should be represented on the root cause analysis team that investigates this patient incident.

   - Evidence that should be presented to the root cause analysis team.
     - Evidence includes written or verbal testimony, physical evidence, and documents. Be as specific as possible.

   - Three root causes of the wrong procedure error. These should be based on your research and what you learned by reading the sentinel event summary provided with this project. The root causes should be specific to the event described in the summary, not just the common root causes of any type of hospital mistake.

   - Three process changes that would prevent a similar error from occurring at the hospital where the sentinel event occurred. These changes should be based on your research and what you learned by reading the sentinel event summary provided with this project. The recommendations should be specific to the hospital described in the scenario, not general recommendations that could apply to any hospital.

Note: If you are not familiar with the terminology used in the sentinel event summary consult a medical dictionary.

Sentinel Event Summary

Mrs. Alice Johnson, a 67-year-old woman with a head injury is admitted to the hospital for cerebral angiography. She mistakenly was subjected to an invasive cardiac electrophysiology study. Fortunately, an hour into the procedure, it was determined that she was the incorrect patient, the procedure was terminated, and she was returned to her room in stable condition. Mrs. Allyce Johnston, a 77-year-old woman, was supposed to have the cardiac studies.

Here is the sequence of events that led up to Alice Johnson having an unnecessary cardiac electrophysiology study:

- The electrophysiology (EP) lab tech calls Allyce Johnston's nursing unit and states that he is looking for a 77-year-old woman scheduled for EP studies. The nurse on this unit incorrectly tells the EP lab tech that the patient he is looking for is on another unit.

- The nurse on the other unit tells the EP lab tech that the patient is there. In fact, the nurse mistakenly thinks that the EP tech is looking for Alice Johnson, the 67-year-old woman with the head injury.

- The nurse transports Alice Johnson to the EP lab for the cardiac study despite the lack of written or verbal order for the study in her record.

- When Alice Johnson arrives in the EP lab, she objects to having the cardiac study as she had not been told by her physician that such a study was to be done. She is ultimately allowed to speak on the phone with the physician who ordered the study for Allyce Johnston. This physician does not realize he is speaking with the wrong patient and, furthermore, Alice Johnson does not realize she is not speaking to her personal physician. The physician tells Alice Johnson that she had given her verbal consent for the EP study even though she had not.

- The EP technician finds no written consent in Alice Johnson's medical record for the study. He explains the need for implantable cardioverter defibrillator (ICD) and pacemaker (PM) and succeeds in gaining her signature on a consent form that states, "EP study with possible ICD and possible PM placement."

- The physician resident who had been caring for Alice Johnson discovers she is no longer in her room. When the nurse says that Alice Johnson is in the EP lab for a scheduled test, the resident presumes the attending physician had ordered the cardiac study and he drops his questioning.

- The EP lab charge nurse notes a discrepancy in patient names right after the start of the study but chooses not to stop the procedure because it was at a delicate juncture. When the interventional cardiologist determines that an ICD is not required he notices the discrepancy in patient names and terminates the procedure.

11.6   Analyze a Root Cause Analysis Investigation

Description

The Agency for Healthcare Research and Quality sponsors a website where you'll find case summaries and commentaries about adverse events and unsafe situations in various types of healthcare facilities. In this project, you'll search this website, select a case discussion about a sentinel event, summarize the investigation and determine how to measure the success of recommended improvement actions.

Instructions

1. Explore WebM&M (https://psnet.ahrq.gov/Webmm). Select from the case archives a discussion of a specific adverse patient incident. Pick a case that meets the Joint Commission definition of a sentinel event. The case should discuss one harmful incident that occurred in a healthcare facility (not a summary discussion on a safety topic).

2. For the case you select, write a report that includes the following elements:

   a. Title of the case and name of the author(s) of the case discussion

   b. Brief summary of the incident (in your own words)

   c. Root cause(s) of the incident as described by the case discussion author(s)

   d. Actions recommended by the author(s) of the case discussion to prevent a similar event from occurring in the future

   e. Two performance measurements that could be used to evaluate the success of the improvement actions recommended by the author(s). Don't just re-state the recommended improvement actions. You are to list two measurements that could be used to judge whether the actions worked. In other words, did the process get safer? Remember, performance measurements start with phrases like: "percentage of …" "rate of …" "number of …"

Building a Safe Medication Management System

12

12.1 Conduct a Failure Mode and Effects Analysis

Description

A failure mode and effects analysis (FMEA) is an improvement project that involves a systematic assessment of a process to identify the location, cause, and consequences of potential failures. The goal of a FMEA is to eliminate or reduce the chance of process failures. In this project you'll conduct a FMEA of a familiar process.

Instructions

1. Download the answer sheet for this project from the AHIMA student website.
2. Review Figure 12.1 top-down flowchart of the activity of going to work.

   Note: The sub-processes are provided for information only. Your personal experiences may differ somewhat from the example.
3. Use the answer sheet provided for this project to complete a FMEA on the process of going to work.

   - Refer to the process steps that are pre-listed in column one. In column two, list what could go wrong (the potential failures) at each of the process steps. There is space on the form to list two failures (one per row) for each process step.
   - For each failure listed in column two, determine what would happen if the failure occurred (the effect) and record this in column three. Each failure should have an effect recorded.
   - Using the risk assessment matrix provided with the answer sheet, rate the likelihood of each failure you've listed in column two. The likelihood rating is a numeric score, ranging from 1–6. Put the likelihood score for each failure in column four.
   - Using the risk assessment scoring matrix provided with the answer sheet, rate the consequence of each effect you've listed in column three. The consequence rating is an alpha score, ranging from A to D. Put the consequence score for each effect in column five.

Figure 12.1: Top-down flowchart of the steps involved in going to work

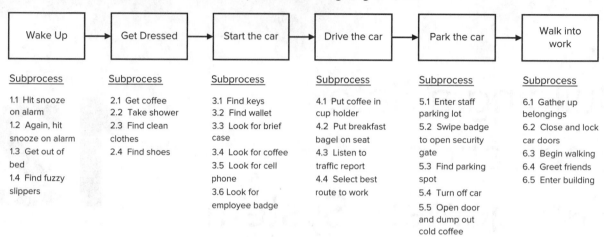

- Using the risk assessment matrix provided with the answer sheet, rate each failure listed in column two as high, medium, or low. This rating is obtained by determining where the frequency and consequence scores for the failure intersect on the matrix. Record the rating for each failure in the last column.

- Select two of the high or medium failures and write a short description of what could be done to prevent each failure from occurring.

Managing the Environment of Care

13

13.1 Investigate an Incident Involving an Unsafe Environment

Description

Root cause analysis is used to evaluate the cause of patient care events with the goal of preventing something similar from occurring. In this case study you'll use root cause analysis to analyze the cause of an environment of care accident, suggest actions to prevent something similar from happening again, and select measures of success.

Instructions

1. Read the case study below:

   A housekeeper who has worked at the hospital for more than five years is waxing the floors near the cafeteria at 1:00 a.m. He cannot find a wet floor sign and would have had to go back to the office to find one. The housekeeping staff frequently must search for wet floor signs which causes them to get behind in their work. Although the manager has been made aware of this problem, no additional signs have been purchased.

   The housekeeper believes there will not be any foot traffic in the area at this time of night, so he does not go to the trouble of finding a sign. Plus, there has not been a problem when he didn't post a sign in the past. He leaves to take his mid-shift break while the floor dries. A young patient, unable to sleep, takes a walk with his mother near the vending machine and slips on the wet floor, breaking his wrist.

2. Create a report that includes the following:

   - Root causes of the event (no more than three or four root causes; dig deeper if you have more than this).
   Note: Root causes are "why" the event occurred, not statements of what happened. A statement of "what happened" is something like: Nurse was rushing. A root cause is "why" this happened, for example, inadequate orientation to the job responsibilities. Given the limited information in the scenario, it is okay to hypothesize the most likely causes.

- Three specific process changes that will be most effective at resolving the root causes and ultimately prevent or greatly reduce the chance the case study event will happen again at the same hospital. Explain each change you are proposing and why you think it will be effective.
- Two performance measurements that can be used to evaluate the success of the process changes you recommend.

Developing Staff and Human Resources

14

14.1　Identify Sources of Physician Performance Expectation Data

Description

In this project you will find some performance data that a hospital medical staff could use to establish physician performance expectations. At the time of reappointment, the hospital medical staff would measure each physician's performance against these expectations. It is very common for health care organizations to use data from other organizations (what other physicians have been able to achieve) to set performance expectations. In this project you will be doing some research to find out what results other organizations have been able to achieve for some specific performance measures. These results can be used to set quantifiable physician performance expectations.

Instructions

1. Download the answer sheet for this project from the AHIMA student website.
2. For each performance measure listed below locate one source that could be used by an organization to establish a performance target. The data should be from a U.S. source and the data should be no more than six years old.

   - Rate of primary caesarean section deliveries
   - Number of medical/surgical intensive care unit (ICU) adult patients who acquire a ventilator-associated pneumonia in the ICU (per 1000 ventilator days)
   - Percent of heart attack patients prescribed a beta-blocker when discharged from the hospital
   - Negative appendectomy rate (percent of patients undergoing appendectomy for infected appendix and the pathology report reveals a normal appendix)
   - Percent of patients developing deep vein thrombosis after hip surgery
   - Percent of patients receiving home health care after a hospitalization who are re-hospitalized within 30 days of the first home health visit.

An example of what the completed project should look like is shown in figure 14.1. You'll be filling in column two of the table on the answer sheet.

You are to list the title of the source in column 2 of the answer sheet along with the exact URL of the website where the source is located.

Figure 14.1: Example of exercise 14.1 step 2

Measure	A Source of information that could be used as a basis for establishing a performance target
Inpatient mortality rate following open heart surgery (includes procedures such as coronary artery bypass surgery and cardiac valve procedures)	Report of cardiac care outcomes in Virginia Hospitals http://www.vhi.org/Cardiac/statewide.asp

3. The source should be publicly available performance data from a credible source. The source must contain some information about what rates are expected or what other organizations have been able to achieve. Sources that merely describe the measure (without any actual performance data) do not serve as a basis for establishing a performance expectation.

Tip: Everything you need is available online. Resources like PubMed (www.ncbi.nlm.nih.gov/pubmed/) will be helpful to you.

14.2 Select Cases for Physician Peer Review

Description

To evaluate professional practices, the hospital medical staff conducts peer review. This involves evaluating the care provided to an individual patient to identify improvement opportunities. Cases selected for peer review are often identified through retrospective record review. The medical staff defines patient care events or situations that signal the need for closer examination of the case. In this project you'll review descriptions of inpatient hospitalizations to identify cases in which one or more of these events or situations occurred.

Instructions

1. Download the answer sheet for this project from the AHIMA student website.

2. Presume you are a data analyst in the hospital health information management department. One of your job responsibilities is to review all records of discharged patients to determine if specific events or situations, known as occurrences, took place a patient's hospital stay. If one or more of the occurrences took place, the case will undergo peer review by members of the medical staff professional practice committee. This committee has requested that you notify it of cases in which one or more of the following events or situations occurred during the patient's hospital stay. Take note of the numbers corresponding to each occurrence. You'll use them later to complete the project.

   01 Cardiac and/or pulmonary arrest, resuscitation successful
   02 Cardiac and/or pulmonary arrest, resuscitation unsuccessful
   03 Cardiac and/or pulmonary arrest, not resuscitated, recovered
   04 Cardiac and/or pulmonary arrest, not resuscitated, expired
   05 Readmission within 30 days for same/similar diagnosis

06 Unplanned admission following outpatient procedure

07 Unplanned return to the operating room

08 Unexpected neurological deficit developed after invasive procedure

09 Renal and/or cardiovascular complications following invasive procedure

10 Reintubation within 24 hours of anesthesia

11 No definitive diagnosis within 72 hours of admission

12 Pathological diagnosis does not match preoperative diagnosis

13 Reports or tests misread or misidentified

14 Extended post-anesthesia recovery unit stay (more than 3 hours)

15 Unplanned transfer to cardiac care unit (CCU) or intensive care unit (ICU)

16 Patient suicide – attempted or successful

17 Admission evening prior to elective surgery without appropriate indications

18 Medication error or adverse drug event resulting in patient injury

19 Patient fall resulting in patient injury

20 Patient discharged "against medical advice"

21 Unplanned removal, injury or repair of an organ or structure during invasive procedure

22 Nosocomial infection

23 Blood transfusion reaction

3. Read the 15 case scenarios that accompany the project.

4. Use the answer sheet provided for the project to identify which (if any) of the events or situations described above actually happened in each of the cases. In the space provided on the answer sheet, record the number to the left of the occurrence. If more than one occurrence happened in a case, record all the relevant occurrence numbers in the space provided. If none of the occurrences happened for a particular case, record zero.

5. After completing the answer sheet, create a data table or graphic report that shows the total number of cases reviewed and the number of occurrences found in each category.

Note: If you are not familiar with the terminology used in the occurrence statements or the case scenarios, consult a medical dictionary.

Case Scenarios

Case 1: An eight-year-old male was seen in the pediatric outpatient clinic on 6/23 complaining of acute abdominal pain. Physical examination and blood tests suggested the patient may have an acute appendicitis and he was immediately transported to the hospital. Upon admission, the patient underwent a C-T scan of the abdomen but it did not show an acute appendicitis. The patient was started on IV antibiotics but his condition failed to improve. The next day, on 6/24 he was taken to surgery with the preoperative diagnosis of "probable acute appendicitis." An appendectomy was performed. The patient's post-operative course was uneventful and he was discharged on 6/25. Pathological examination of the appendix revealed no inflammation. The patient's final diagnosis, as documented by the surgeon, was "acute bacterial gastroenteritis."

Case 2: On 4/11, a 68-year-old male patient was admitted to the intensive care unit at the hospital with diagnoses that included congestive heart failure, non-insulin dependent diabetes, edema of the lower extremities with cellulitis, ulcer of his toe, hypertension, and bladder outlet obstruction. On 4/13 he underwent a non-invasive vascular study procedure. Following the procedure, the patient suffered a cardiac arrest. Caregivers started cardiopulmonary resuscitation immediately, however, the resuscitation attempts failed. The attending physician documented that the patient's death was due to complications of severe congestive heart failure secondary to cardiovascular disease.

Case 3: On 6/15, a 53-year-old female was admitted to the hospital for surgical repair of a broken left fibula, sustained at home when she fell out of her wheelchair. Her medical history included diabetes, chronic kidney failure, thyroid, and pulmonary problems. She had the surgery on 6/16 and was given two units of blood during surgery. Postoperatively she had problems with hyperglycemia. The patient's condition eventually stabilized, and she was discharged to a skilled nursing facility for continued physical therapy on 6/27.

Case 4: On 3/23 a 32-year-old female underwent a planned C-section at the hospital. She also had a tubal ligation at the same time. For several weeks after the procedure, she had gastrointestinal complaints and chronic diarrhea and was seen by her primary care physician and a gastroenterologist. Two months after her C-section she presented to your hospital emergency department with acute abdominal pain, thought due to a bowel obstruction. A CT scan at that time showed a retained sponge from her previous C-section and tubal ligation surgery. During her second hospitalization she underwent surgery for removal of the sponge and repair of a perforated bowel.

Case 5: On 6/24, a 70-year-old woman was admitted to the medical unit of the hospital following an extensive stroke that left her with a swallowing disorder. On admission a soft, small-diameter (10 French) nasogastric feeding tube was inserted into the patient's stomach by her physician. The correct location of the tube was confirmed by auscultation. Two hours after admission, a nurse gave the patient a pint of enteral feeding supplement through the tube. Thirty minutes later, the nurse noticed the patient was cyanotic and having difficulty breathing. The patient's physician was contacted, and the patient was transferred to the intensive care unit. A chest x-ray revealed that the feeding tube was in the lower lobe of the patient's right lung and not in the correct location in the stomach. The patient developed aspiration pneumonia following this incident and ultimately expired on 6/25. Respecting the patient's "Do Not Resuscitate" request, the caregivers did not attempt cardiopulmonary resuscitation.

Case 6: On 4/11, a 68-year-old male patient was transferred to the hospital from another facility for a non-invasive outpatient procedure. The patient's diagnoses included congestive heart failure, non-insulin dependent diabetes, edema of the lower extremities with cellulitis, ulcer of his toe, hypertension, and bladder outlet obstruction. The patient's medical records from the transferring hospital were sent along with the patient and were available to physicians prior to the procedure. The patient had been receiving oxygen at one liter per minute at the transferring facility and during transport but after admission to your hospital the patient did not receive oxygen because it was not ordered at the time of his admission. The patient underwent the non-invasive vascular study procedure on 4/13. Following the procedure, the patient suffered a seizure and a cardiac arrest. Caregivers started cardiopulmonary resuscitation immediately however continued resuscitation attempts failed. The attending physician documented that the patient's death was due to complications of severe congestive heart failure secondary to cardiovascular disease.

Case 7: On 6/17 an 84-year-old female, admitted to the hospital for pneumonia and chronic obstructive lung disease, was found by staff on the floor by her bed. The patient was assessed and found to have a laceration on her nose with some bleeding from that area. She also had a bruise on the right shoulder. The patient's physician was notified. Four hours later, a staff nurse noted the patient had a swelling and bruising of the right wrist. The patient's physician was notified again and an x-ray was ordered. The x-ray revealed a questionable non-displaced fracture of the wrist which was treated with an ace-wrap. The nursing staff placed a bed alarm on the patient's bed after this occurrence and no further patient falls occurred. The patient was discharged to home care on 6/25. The home health agency was notified that the patient is at high-risk for future falls and a home safety assessment was recommended.

Case 8: A 36-year-old male patient had elective knee surgery at the hospital on 6/09. The patient had no apparent intraoperative or postoperative complications until he complained of shortness of breath and chest pain at approximately 6:00 p.m. on 6/11. The orthopedic surgeon assessed the patient, moved him to the intensive care unit and obtained a cardiology consult. The cardiologist assessed the patient and determined that the patient's problems were not cardiac related. A pulmonologist consultation was obtained and a pulmonary scan showed multiple pulmonary emboli. A cardiac surgeon was asked to consult in regards to embolectomy surgery. The surgeon did not choose to operate due to the high risk related to the patient's weight (he weighed over 300 pounds). It was decided to treat the emboli conservatively with a heparin drip to dissolve the clots. The drip was started at 8:00 p.m. on 6/11. The patient had cardiac arrest at 12:28 p.m. on 6/12 and all attempts at resuscitation failed. The patient was pronounced dead at 1:28 p.m. The family refused an autopsy and the coroner was not called. Cause of death was noted to be pulmonary embolus.

Case 9: A 59-year-old male was admitted to the hospital on 4/7 for diagnostic studies related to an occluded internal carotid artery, low grade carotid disease and dilated abdominal aorta. While undergoing a carotid arteriogram, he had a cerebrovascular accident and underwent an emergency carotid endarterectomy. His condition deteriorated while in the recovery room following the endarterectomy and he required two units of packed cells. This caused him to remain in the recovery room for more than four hours. The remainder of the patient's hospitalization was uneventful, and he was discharged to home on 4/23.

Case 10: A 39-year-old male was admitted to the hospital's psychiatric care unit on 4/15 for treatment of depression and suicidal ideation. He was given a physical examination on the day of his admission; however, there was a three-day delay in drawing his blood for routine lab work. When these results did return, they showed a very high blood glucose level, as did additional tests. By this time the treatment team had determined the patient was ready for discharge so the treating psychiatrist, believing the patient needed evaluation of what was likely diabetes, developed a discharge plan that included an immediate outpatient evaluation by the patient's primary care physician. The patient was discharged on 4/27. Twenty-five days later, the patient, who never went to see his primary care physician, was re-admitted to the hospital with severe hyperglycemia. After 48 hours in the hospital, the patient's diabetic condition stabilized. He was started on insulin and received diabetic education and nutritional counseling. The patient was eventually discharged to home on 6/8. His physician ordered a few weeks of home health services to help reinforce what the patient had learned in the hospital.

Case 11: On 4/23, a 56-year-old female patient in the hospital was getting a pre-surgery antibiotic by intravenous injection when she developed a rash and vomited. The patient's nurse stopped the intravenous antibiotic as soon as the patient experienced difficulties. The patient quickly became unresponsive and had a respiratory arrest. Cardiopulmonary resuscitation was successful. The patient was transferred to the intensive care unit and treated for an anaphylactic reaction. The patient did not have a documented allergy to the antibiotic prior to this hospitalization. The patient's condition stabilized, and she was discharged home on 5/1. Her surgery was scheduled for a later date.

Case 12: On 5/3, a 62-year-old male in the hospital for chemotherapy treatments was found lying at the foot of the stairs in the north wing stairwell (a back exit intended for use by staff only). The patient told the nurse who found him that he had fallen down the stairs. The nurse assessed the patient and found no apparent injury. She helped the patient return to his room. A later examination by his physician revealed minor bruising but no other injuries. Upon investigation, it was found that the alarm on the door to the stairwell had been repaired earlier in the day and the alarm had not been reset. That was why staff was not alerted when the patient opened the door to the stairwell. The patient had no ill effects from the fall and he was discharged home on 5/7.

Case 13: On 5/18 a 35-year-old, female patient in your hospital's psychiatric unit failed to return from an authorized six-hour off-site pass. The physician and responsible medical staff were notified of the elopement. Attempts made to reach the patient using the telephone number supplied by the patient were unsuccessful. The patient had been assessed and was found not to be a risk to herself or others at the time the pass was issued, however her physician did not yet feel she was ready to be discharged from inpatient care at the time she was given the pass. Discharge procedures were begun on 5/20 when she still had failed to return.

Case 14: On 5/13, a 36-year-old intoxicated male was admitted to the hospital's detoxification unit. Approximately two hours after admission, the patient became violent and as staff intervened, the patient struck the staff member in the face. Facility security and the police department were called. The patient was arrested by the police and transported to jail on charges of assault.

Case 15: A 46-year-old female was admitted to the hospital on 4/15 for an abdominal hysterectomy. Three days after her initial operation, the patient complained of abdominal pain. The pain did not subside and on the sixth day, her gynecologist did exploratory surgery. At the time of surgery, the doctor discovered that a portion of patient's bowel had slipped through a small hole in the membrane covering her abdomen. This defect, which occurred during the first surgery, was repaired and the patient was transferred to the intensive care unit postoperatively. The next day, the patient had a 103.8° F fever and her urine output sharply declined. A third surgery was performed to remove six feet of necrotic bowel. The patient went downhill rapidly and within 24 hours following the second bowel surgery, she was placed on mechanical ventilation. The patient ultimately developed a septic bacterial infection and kidney failure. Despite aggressive treatment and two more abdominal surgeries, the patient expired on 6/25 secondary to multiple organ failure. The family had requested that the patient not be resuscitated.

14.3   Measure Non-Licensed Staff Member Competence

Description

Healthcare organizations have the legal responsibility to ensure the competence of all licensed and non-licensed full-time and part-time employees. To fulfill this responsibility employers periodically evaluate everyone's ability to satisfactorily perform their job. In this project you'll identify measures of employee performance based on their defined job responsibilities.

Instructions

1. Read the job description for the Health System Database Analyst provided with this project.
2. Considering the job responsibilities and skill requirements for the Database Analyst, list at least five measures of performance that could be utilized to judge this individual's continued competence.
3. For each performance measure indicate where information to evaluate this aspect of the individual's performance could be found.

Job Description for Health System Database Analyst

Primary Function: Design, implement, and modify database systems; analyze user data requirements; monitor the performance of production databases; provide assistance to users.

Major Duties and Responsibilities:

- Design, implement, and modify database systems.
- Analyze user data requirements and determine database usage and required hardware and software support
- Determine access methods and compatibility with overall database system
- Develop database standards/procedures; design forms and reports
- Monitor production database performance and make necessary changes to improve performance
- Compile data and write reports and letters
- Update data dictionary
- Provide technical assistance to users
- Perform computer studies and operates computer equipment

- Keep up-to-date on database techniques, systems, and programming technology
- Perform other duties as assigned

Supervisory Responsibility: As a project leader, supervise systems analyst, programmers, and other data processing staff. Instruct in methods and procedures and may assign work and establish priorities or make recommendations regarding discipline and employee problems.

Budgetary Responsibility: In conjunction with other employees, is indirectly responsible for the development, implementation, and control of departmental budget.

Communications

Internal: Frequent contact with data processing staff and various levels of staff and faculty in other departments to exchange information on design requirements and schedules and to solve user problems.
External: Occasional contact with vendor representatives related to the purchase of their products.
Patient Contact: No contact with patients.

Physical Requirements

Requires regular, moderate physical effort. Eyestrain and stress from meeting deadlines.

Working Environment

Seldom or never exposed to unpleasant working conditions.

Job Specifications

Education/Experience: Skills and knowledge are normally acquired through completion of a bachelor's degree in computer science or related field. A minimum of four years of experience in database design and planning, including two years of systems development experience at a project leader level.

Licensure/Certification: No licensure or certification required.

Job-related Skills: Thorough knowledge of computer technology, programming, practices, procedures, equipment, and languages used in computer operation. Numerical ability sufficient to program at level of linear and Boolean algebra and differential equations. Thorough knowledge of statistical analysis.

Organizing and Evaluating Performance Improvement

15

15.1   Document Medical Staff Peer Review Results

Description

Professional practice evaluations are an important component of hospital medical staff quality management responsibilities. One element of this evaluation involves individual case review. In this project you'll create a form to be used to gather information about cases needing review by the medical staff and a form that can be used by physicians to document the case review findings.

Instructions

1. Read the "Anesthesia Department Quality Management Plan" provided with this project.
2. Design a one-page form, known as the anesthesia occurrence form, that can be used for step 1 of the case review process (described under the heading "Case Reviews" in the Quality Management Plan).
3. Develop a case review form that can be used by physicians to document results of their in-depth case review process (described in steps 5 and 6 of the case review process).

Anesthesia Department Quality Management Plan

Purpose

The purpose of this plan is to define the format within which the Anesthesia Department carries out its Quality Management Program.

Scope and Responsibility

The anesthesiology department is comprised of anesthesiologists and certified registered nurse anesthetists (CRNAs) who are responsible for all anesthesia services provided anywhere in the hospital. The chair of anesthesia is responsible for maintaining quality patient care services in the department. To assure that the care provided is in accordance with recognized standards of practice, the anesthesiology department has an ongoing professional practice evaluation system which incorporates concurrent surveillance, objective performance assessment, and meaningful continuing education with appropriate credentialing. The chair of anesthesia is responsible for assuring that this program is carried out effectively. Day-to-day activities of surveillance, performance assessment, and education are delegated to the anesthesia quality management committee.

Evaluation Methodology

All care provided by the department is regularly evaluated by the department's quality management committee utilizing performance measures and peer review of individual cases. On a quarterly basis, the hospital quality department provides the chief of anesthesia with individual practitioner profiles that include volume of cases, performance measure results, number of cases selected for in-depth peer review, and the peer review results.

Performance Measures

At least quarterly, the committee reviews performance data for the following measures:

- Percent of patients whose perioperative serum glucose was maintained at or below 200 mg/dl during cardiac surgery
- Percent of patients receiving appropriate perioperative prophylaxis for venous thromboembolism
- Percent of patients on mechanical ventilation that have head of bed elevated
- Percent of patients on mechanical ventilation that followed appropriate weaning protocol in postoperative period
- Percent of patients experiencing a minor or moderate event during surgery (for example, cut or blistered tongue, loosened or chipped tooth, etc.)
- Percent of surgery delays attributable to anesthesia
- Percent of surgery patient records with documentation of pre-anesthesia evaluation by anesthesiologist or CRNA
- Percent of surgery patient records with documentation of post-anesthesia evaluation by anesthesiologist or CRNA

Case Reviews

The Quality Management Committee regularly reviews cases in which one or more of the following events occurred:

- Surgery cancelled after anesthetic induction
- Significant perioperative injury to patient attributable to anesthesia
- Major break in aseptic technique attributable to anesthesia
- Anesthesia equipment or instrumentation problem any time during surgery
- Patient has temperature below 93.2°F in post-anesthesia recovery unit
- Cardiac or respiratory arrest (during surgery or in post-anesthesia recovery unit)

- Death in preoperative, intraoperative, or postoperative areas
- Patient discharged from post-anesthesia recovery unit without meeting discharge criteria
- Patient has allergic reaction to anesthesia agent
- Patient leaves operating room or post-anesthesia recovery unit on unplanned ventilator or intubation
- Unplanned hospital admission following outpatient surgery/procedure
- Anesthetized patient experiences intraoperative awareness
- Clinically apparent acute myocardial infarction within forty-eight hours of anesthesia
- Development of post-dural puncture headache within twenty-four hours of anesthesia.
- Aspiration gastric contents with development of aspiration pneumonia within twenty-four hours of anesthesia.
- Other anesthesia-related complications (corneal abrasion, pulmonary edema, laryngospasm, postoperative delirium)

In addition to the above events, potential cases for peer review are also identified by several other means, for example, department of health reports, referrals from risk management, patient incident reports, and patient/family complaints. Regardless of the source, the case review process remains the same.

The case review process is described below.

1. An anesthesia occurrence form is provided to the circulating nurse upon each patient's entry to the operating suite holding area and is collected by the nurse in the recovery area when the patient is discharged. Throughout the surgical/obstetrical experience, any reviewable occurrence or other miscellaneous deviations from the norm are documented by the circulating or recovery nurse on the occurrence form.

2. The completed occurrence forms are forwarded to the hospital quality department where they are reviewed. Cases identified as relevant to the anesthesia review process are copied and entered into the Anesthesia professional practice evaluation database. All records (with or without occurrences) have basic data entered into the database to obtain accurate denominator information.

3. In addition to the above process, potential events for case review identified by other means are entered into the professional practice evaluation database.

4. The first step of the case review process is carried out by the members of the anesthesia quality management committee. All cases in which a reviewable event occurred are summarized by quality department staff and the information is forwarded, on a rotating basis, to the members of the committee. This first review is made to determine if, in fact, the event was anesthesia related. No further action is necessary on those cases deemed not anesthesia related, except possible referral to another medical staff service or hospital department if deemed appropriate.

5. Those events found to be anesthesia-related undergo evaluation of the case by members of the anesthesia quality management committee. This in-depth peer review process includes an analysis of the following issues:

- Soundness of practitioner's judgment
- Adherence to safe practices
- Adequacy of preoperative preparation of the patient for anesthesia and operation
- Proper intraoperative patient management
- Proper pharmacological management
- Recognition and response to significant changes in the patient's intraoperative anesthetic course
- Provision of appropriate post-anesthetic care
- Appropriate and timely documentation of anesthesia-related patient care

The attending anesthesiologist may be contacted in writing, requesting his or her input in answering questions or providing undocumented information. The results of the case review process are documented on the review form. Cases may be deemed acceptable or the quality of the clinical management and/or documentation may be questioned. These findings are documented on the anesthesia case review form, in the committee's minutes, and added to the case file in the professional practice evaluation database.

6. If cases are found to be unacceptable the Committee's recommendations are presented at the weekly Departmental meetings where they are thoroughly discussed, and final decisions rendered regarding the quality of care and adequacy of documentation.

7. The attending anesthesiologist will be notified of any cases found to be unacceptable and offered the opportunity to appeal the decision according to the appeals process established in the medical staff bylaws.

8. Final decisions made at the weekly departmental meetings are entered into the case file in the professional practice evaluation database. Case summaries of unacceptable cases are placed into the relevant individual's credentialing files and maintained for later practice pattern analysis.

9. On a quarterly basis, the quality department provides the chief of anesthesia with individual practitioner profiles that include volume of cases, performance measure results, number of cases selected for in-depth peer review, and the peer review results.

15.2   Role of Hospital Managers in Quality and Patient Safety

Description

The board and senior managers in healthcare organizations play an important role in assuring quality care is continually delivered to patients. While the article you'll read is about hospitals, the principles covered apply to any healthcare setting.

Instructions

1. Obtain the article: Parand, A., Dopson, S., Renz, A., and Vincent, C. 2014. "The Role of Hospital Managers in Quality and Patient Safety: A Systematic Review." *BMJ open*, 4(9). Your instructor may provide you with a copy of the article or it can be found online at: https://www.ncbi.nlm.nih.gov/pmc/articles/PMC4158193/.

2. Read the article and identify key points. Circling these points will help you find them when you write. Write notes in the margin and use a highlighter to mark important sections. Talk about the article with others and see if you can explain it to somebody who has not read it. Spend about half your work time for this assignment on this step.

3. Write a summary of the article. The summary should be 400 words or the word length may be set by your instructor. At a minimum, the summary should include the following:

   • Description of the research study, including the study methodology
   • Study results and its contribution toward answering these questions:
      ○ What specific board and senior management practices do not appear to contribute to high quality patient care?
      ○ What specific board and senior management practices do appear to contribute to high quality patient care?

Navigating the Accreditation, Certification, or Licensure Process

16

16.1 Create Plan to Evaluate Compliance with Accreditation Requirements

Description

Presume you work at a nursing care facility accredited by the Joint Commission. The quality department has asked you to develop a plan to evaluate facility-wide compliance with the Joint Commission's national patient safety goals.

Instructions

1. Read the current Joint Commission national patient safety goals for nursing care facilities found online at https://www.jointcommission.org/standards/national-patient-safety-goals /nursing-care-center-national-patient-safety-goals/.

2. Write a memo to the quality department describing how you will determine whether the nursing care facility is complying with each of the patient safety goals and whether caregivers are following the requirements. Include your sources for evaluating compliance and how you will gather compliance information.

Implementing Effective Information Management Tools for Performance Improvement

17

17.1 Information Technology Contributions to Healthcare Quality

Description

The 2001 Institute of Medicine (IOM) report, *Crossing the Quality Chasm: A New Health System for the 21st Century* identified six key dimensions of healthcare quality that need improving. Health information technology (HIT) plays a role in healthcare quality. In this project, you'll describe to a hospital's quality manager how HIT can contribute to improved performance in the key dimensions identified by the IOM.

Instructions

1. Read the six key dimensions of healthcare quality from the *Crossing the Quality Chasm* report listed below.

   - *Healthcare should be Safe – unintended patient injuries should be avoided.*
   - *Healthcare should be Effective – based on scientific knowledge, service should be provided* to all who could benefit. Services should not be provided to people who are not likely to benefit. We should avoid underuse of services as well as overuse.
   - *Healthcare should be Patient-Centered – this means* providing care that is respectful of and responsive to individual patient preferences, needs, and values and ensuring that patient values guide all clinical decisions.
   - *Healthcare should be Timely – we should* reduce waits and sometimes harmful delays for those who receive care.
   - *Healthcare should be Efficient – we should* avoid waste, including waste of equipment, supplies, ideas, and energy.

- *Healthcare should be Equitable – this means that healthcare* should not vary in quality because of a patient's personal characteristics such as gender, ethnicity, geographic location, and socioeconomic status. (Source: Institute of Medicine, Committee on Quality of Health Care in America. *Crossing the Quality Chasm: A New Health System for the 21st Century.* 2001. Washington (DC): National Academies Press).

2. Research how HIT has already or is expected to contribute to improving performance in each key dimension of healthcare quality. A good resource for this research is the ONC website: https://www.healthit.gov.

3. Write a report for the hospital quality manager that summarizes your research findings. Include your references. To complete this report, use the following definition of health information technology: "The application of information processing involving both computer hardware and software that deals with the storage, retrieval, sharing, and use of health care information, data, and knowledge for communication and decision making." (Source: The U.S. Department of Health & Human Services' Office of the National Coordinator for Health IT [ONC] www.healthit.gov/topic /health-it-and-health-information-exchange-basics/glossary).

17.2 Measure Compliance with Practice Guidelines Using EHR Data

Description

With most health clinics now having electronic health records (EHRs), gathering data for measurement projects can be easier, yet challenges remain. In this project you'll research the advantages and challenges of using an EHR to gather data for a study.

Background

Presume you are the quality manager in a 10-physician internal medicine and family practice clinic. The clinic has maintained EHRs for several years. The clinic's medical director requests that a study be done to examine physician practices when treating patients with group A streptococcal (GAS) pharyngitis. The purpose of the study is to identify possible underuse or overuse of throat cultures or rapid strep tests for confirming the diagnosis and examine the appropriateness of antibiotic prescriptions.

The director wants all the records of patients seen in the past year in the clinic with the diagnosis of pharyngitis due to GAS to be reviewed. He provides a recently published clinical practice guideline on the topic of treating patients who present with symptoms of pharyngitis. The quality manager must use the guideline recommendations to evaluate use of throat cultures, rapid strep tests, and antibiotic prescribing among clinic physicians.

Instructions

1. Use data from the clinic's electronic health record system to complete the study. For each case will collect demographic information about the patient, for example, age, sex, race, and the name of the patient's treating physician. In addition, answer the following questions:

   - Did the patient have a throat culture at the first clinic visit?
   - Did the patient's condition meet high-risk criteria for which an immediate throat culture is indicated?
   - Did the patient have a rapid strep screen at the first clinic visit?

- Did the patient's condition meet signs/symptoms for GAS for which a rapid strep screen is indicated?
- Did the patient's condition warrant treatment with an antibiotic?
- If the patient was prescribed an antibiotic, was it a preferred antibiotic treatment regimen?

2. Write a report that addresses the following:

- Advantages of using the clinic's EHR system to gather data for this pharyngitis study.
- Challenges associated with using the clinic's EHR system to collect valid and reliable information for this pharyngitis study.

3. Cite at least two scholarly references to support your responses. These must be in addition to any references you may cite for books or articles that you've been assigned to read for this course.

17.3 Use Publicly Available Performance Data to Judge Healthcare Quality

Description

Among national efforts to improve the quality of healthcare, perhaps none has been as prominent as the movement to evaluate healthcare quality and disclose results of that evaluation publicly, usually in the form of report cards, provider profiles, or consumer reports—sometimes communicated via the Internet. The purpose of public disclosure of information on quality is twofold: to facilitate informed choice and to stimulate quality improvement. In this project you'll use publicly available performance measurement data to make an informed choice among providers.

Background

Presume that your maternal grandfather, who lives just down the block from you, needs to go to a nursing home. Your mother has asked you to help her make the best choice of a nursing home for her father, who has Alzheimer's disease. Her father has Medicare insurance but does not qualify for Medicaid coverage currently.

Instructions

1. Use the resources and information found on the Medicare provider compare website (https://www. medicare.gov/care-compare/) to find nursing homes located no more than 50 miles from your location. Using the data available on the site, recommend two nursing homes for your grandfather and two nursing homes for him to avoid.

2. Write a letter to your mother detailing the information you found. For each nursing home explain the performance factors you considered (services, quality measure results, inspection reports, staffing, and the like) and why you are making the recommendations (in favor of the home or against the home). The factors you consider should be based *only* on information that is available on the Medicare website. At a minimum, consider both the quality measure results and the inspection reports for the nursing homes you recommend and for those you don't recommend.

Tips: Include the actual names of the nursing homes in the letter to your mother and the *exact* performance factors you used to make your judgments. You should have objective and measurable reasons for recommending or not recommending a particular nursing home. For instance, don't recommend a nursing home with a high number of inspection deficiencies just because it is non-profit or because it accepts Medicare patients. Don't recommend against a nursing home just because of its location or its bed size. Use the information on the site to make informed decisions. Don't make assumptions or express opinions without performance data to back them up.

17.4   Overcoming eMeasure Data Collection Barriers

Description

Data for eMeasures are obtained exclusively from electronic health records (EHRs) and/or health information technology systems. In this project you'll explore common barriers to gathering accurate measurement data from EHRs and discuss strategies for overcoming these barriers.

Instructions

1. Download the report, "Capturing High Quality Electronic Health Records Data to Support Performance Improvement" published by The Office of the National Coordinator for Health Information Technology in July 2013. A PDF copy of the report can be obtained at: https://www.healthit.gov/sites/default /files/onc-beacon-lg3-ehr-data-quality-and-perform-impvt.pdf

2. Read the section in the report entitled "Confirm Ability to Extract Data from EHR for Reporting Purposes" (pages 21-24).

3. In your own words summarize barriers to extracting data for measurement purposes from EHRs and strategies for overcoming these barriers. Find at least two other literature references to support your comments.

Managing Healthcare Performance Improvement Projects

18

18.1 Charter a Performance Improvement Project

Description

When an opportunity for improvement is identified, an improvement project is initiated. Ideally, the leadership group or manager originating the project creates a written project charter. The project charter is a condensed, summary-level overview of the project that defines the scope and objectives of the improvement initiative, as well as identifies the departments or individuals who will be involved. In this project you'll create a charter for a multidisciplinary improvement project.

Background: Description of Hospital Nosocomial Infection Problem

Mr. Walker, a 65-year-old male patient has a history of complicated diverticulitis that resulted in a temporary colostomy. He underwent reversal surgery at City Center Hospital (CCH). His recovery on the surgical unit was uneventful and he was soon discharged home. After resuming a normal diet, Mr. Walker continued to have discomfort in his lower abdomen and he then developed very frequent watery diarrhea. When he found blood in his stool, Mr. Walker decided to go to the emergency department where he reported to the nurses that he felt like he "has to sit on the toilet all day." Mr. Walker was readmitted to the surgical unit at CCH for further workup and treatment for probable *Clostridium difficile* (*C. diff*) infection.

Kate Pederson, an infection control practitioner at CCH, was alerted to Mr. Walker's readmission for treatment of an infection he most likely picked up during his first hospitalization. Kate had recently noticed a spike in hospital acquired *C. diff* infections. Nine cases were identified in the past 8 weeks on the same surgical unit where Mr. Walker underwent reversal surgery and recovery.

C. diff infections is a prevalent hospital acquired infection. Most cases occur in patients who have taken or are currently taking antibiotics, who have long hospital stays, colon surgery, or are immune compromised. *C. diff* forms spores that resist drying, heat, pressure, and many disinfectants. Spores can live up to 5 months on solid surfaces such as bed rails, TV controls, equipment, door knobs, and bathroom fixtures. In addition, spores can dwell on the hands of just about anyone entering the hospital environment including providers, patients, family members, house keepers, volunteers, students, and other visitors. Preventing the spread of *C. diff* requires careful attention to environmental cleaning, rigorous hand hygiene, and antibiotic prescribing.

The hospital infection control committee wants Kate to lead a team of people who will conduct a *C. diff* prevention project. Presume you are a member of this committee.

Instructions

Write a project charter for this team by answering the questions below:

- What is the aim of project? Describe what the committee wants the team to accomplish.
- How will success be measured? Identify at least three process or outcome measures.
- Who should be on the team? Identify the groups or departments that should be represented on the team.

Managing the Human Side of Change

19

19.1 Conduct a Force Field Analysis

Description

A force field analysis is a way for an improvement team to identify "driving" (positive) forces and "restraining" (negative) forces for a proposed plan of action. As an example, if a team of climbers headed for the peak of Mt. Everest were to do a force field analysis it might look like this:

Driving Forces   **Restraining Forces**
Good equipment   *The cold*
Maps and charts   *Thin air (difficulty breathing)*
Past climbing experience   *Dangers (falling, etc.)*

A force field helps an improvement team evaluate the possible strengths of negative and positive forces and decide what can be done to maximize the driving forces and minimize the restraining ones. In this case study you'll conduct a force field analysis.

Instructions

1. Obtain a force field analysis template from your instructor or download one from: http://www .findwordtemplates.com/force-field-analysis-templates.html.

2. Complete a force field analysis for a personal plan – that is, take a professional certification exam offered by an organization. Pick an exam for which you are (or will be) eligible to take. Record the name of the exam in the space provided for "desired state" or "plan" on the force field analysis template you downloaded.

3. Using the force field analysis template on the answer sheet, list at least five "driving" (positive) forces for taking the certification exam and at least five "restraining" (negative) forces.

4. Write a report that describes what you can do to maximize the driving forces and minimize the restraining ones.

Understanding the Legal Implications of Performance Improvement

20

20.1 Evaluate Compliance with Institutional Adverse Event Disclosure Policy

Description

The Joint Commission requires that patients are told when an adverse event has occurred during provision of care. An adverse event necessitating such disclosure: "has a perceptible effect on the patient that was not discussed in advance as a known risk; necessitates a change in the patient's care; potentially poses an important risk to the patient's future health," even if the risk is small; or "involves providing a treatment or procedure without the patient's consent" (Cantor et al. 2005). In this case study you'll review the disclosure policy of a healthcare facility and identify how to measure compliance with the policy.

Instructions

1. Read the policy memorandum regarding disclosure of adverse events at South Texas Veterans Health Care System. This policy can be found online at: https://www.uthscsa.edu/sites/default/files/2018/va_disclosure_of_adverse_events_policy.pdf.

2. Write a report describing how the risk manager can measure whether caregivers at the hospital are complying with the policy.

Bonus Case Studies

B.1 Elements of a Successful Quality Management Effort

Description

Continuous quality improvement in healthcare organizations requires a planned and systematic approach. In this project you'll learn the important elements of a successful healthcare quality management approach at the organization and at the department level.

Instructions

1. Read the forward in this book.
2. Considering the information found in the forward, write a report for the director of a hospital health information management (HIM) department that includes the following topics:

   - The four elements, according to the forward, that must be in place for an organization to achieve quality.
   - The internal and external customers of the HIM department in a hospital
   - Processes in the HIM department that are most important to customers
   - The best way to improve processes in the HIM department so customers will be better satisfied with the output
   - Those responsible for improving the quality of services in the HIM department.

B.2 Quality-of-Life Measurement Instruments

Description

Survey instruments are often used to gather information from patients about their general health status and health-related quality of life. These surveys ask people questions about their physical functioning, social functioning, role functioning, mental health, and general health perceptions (for example, vitality, pain, cognitive functioning). In this project you'll identify sources of quality-of-life survey instruments and describe the quality dimensions being measured by the surveys.

Background

Presume you are the quality manager at a large orthopedic clinic. The medical director wants to measure the quality of life for patients with back pain that are being treated conservatively (no surgical procedures). The director wants to send a survey to these patients to measure their quality of life at six and twelve months following their first clinic visit for treatment of back pain.

Instructions

1. Conduct research to identify two measurement instruments that could be used to measure the quality of life for patients with back pain who are being treated conservatively.

2. For each instrument, specify the name of the developer and the various quality-of-life dimensions that the instrument measures.

B.3 Using IOM Quality Dimensions to Identify Improvement Projects

Description

The Institute of Medicine (IOM) six key dimensions of healthcare quality is a good starting point for identifying improvement project opportunities. In this case study you'll apply these dimensions to an actual healthcare experience you or someone you know has had.

Instructions

1. Think about an experience you, a family member, or a friend has had with healthcare facility. Compare this experience to the IOM's six dimensions of healthcare performance (listed below) to identify improvement opportunities.

   - Healthcare should be Safe – unintended patient injuries should be avoided.

   - Healthcare should be Effective – based on scientific knowledge, service should be provided to all who could benefit. Services should not be provided to people who are not likely to benefit. We should avoid underuse of services as well as overuse.

   - Healthcare should be Patient-Centered – this means providing care that is respectful of and responsive to individual patient preferences, needs, and values and ensuring that patient values guide all clinical decisions.

- Healthcare should be Timely – we should reduce waits and sometimes harmful delays for those who receive care.
- Healthcare should be Efficient – we should avoid waste, including waste of equipment, supplies, ideas, and energy.
- Healthcare should be Equitable – this means that healthcare should not vary in quality because of a patient's personal characteristics such as gender, ethnicity, geographic location, and socioeconomic status. (Source: Committee on Quality of Health Care in America, Institute of Medicine. 2001. *Crossing the Quality Chasm: A New Health System for the 21st Century*. Washington (DC): National Academies Press).

2. Write a report that describes:
   a. How the healthcare experience meets or does not meet each quality dimension. Consider questions such as: Was the facility's approach to care patient centered? How safe did you/they feel while receiving care? How effective was the care you/they received? Was the care provided in an efficient and timely manner? Would the treatment you/they received be available to low-income patients?
   b. After applying IOM's six quality dimensions discuss how these insights may be used by managers in a healthcare facility when selecting quality improvement projects.

B.4   Create and Interpret a Scatter Diagram

Description

A scatter diagram (sometimes called a scatter plot) is a simple visual form of graphical analysis. It can be used by an improvement team to investigate a potential relationship between two performance variables. In this project you'll create a scatter diagram from measurement data and interpret the results.

Instructions

1. Presume you are the quality director in a long-term care facility. You are facilitating a team charged with reducing medication errors. One factor the team thinks may be causing a higher rate of medication errors is staffing. Some of the team members feel strongly that medication errors increase when there are fewer registered nurses (RNs) and licensed practical nurses (LPNs) on duty. To investigate this assumption, you gather data on nurse staffing levels and medication errors for 50 random days. Figure B.1 shows the results of your data collection.

2. Create a scatter diagram that shows the relationship between number of medication errors and number of nursing staff on duty. Plot number of errors on the *y*-axis and number of nurses on duty on the *x*-axis.

3. Write a report that answers the following questions: Were the team members correct in their assumption? Is there a positive relationship between medication errors and the number of nurses on duty? Briefly describe what the scatter diagram reveals.

B.5   Analyze Patient Outcome Data

Description

In this project you'll review two reports of mortality rates for infants in neonatal intensive care units at 17 different hospitals. The mortality rates in one report are risk-adjusted – meaning various patient factors

Figure B.1:   Number of nurses on duty and number of medication errors for 50 day period

Day	Number of nurses on duty	Number of medication errors	Day	Number of nurses on duty	Number of medication errors
1	6	0	26	2	4
2	4	0	27	3	3
3	3	2	28	2	4
4	2	5	29	5	1
5	6	0	30	5	0
6	3	2	31	3	3
7	4	1	32	6	0
8	2	5	33	2	3
9	4	0	34	3	3
10	5	1	35	6	0
11	3	2	36	5	0
12	2	4	37	3	3
13	4	1	38	2	3
14	6	0	39	5	0
15	3	2	40	2	4
16	5	0	41	5	1
17	3	4	42	2	4
18	4	2	43	4	4
19	3	4	44	2	2
20	4	0	45	5	5
21	3	4	46	5	5
22	6	0	47	3	3
23	3	4	48	4	4
24	6	0	49	3	3
25	2	4	50	6	6

influencing mortality rates have been accounted for. The mortality rates in the second report are crude data – meaning that various patient factors influencing mortality rates have not been accounted for. You are to speculate why the two reports, which are from the same time period for the same sites, show different results.

Instructions

Background

Figure B.2 and B.3 are two reports of infant mortality rates at neonatal intensive care units (NICU) at 17 different hospital sites. The mortality rates are risk-adjusted in one report and not risk-adjusted in the other report. The average mortality rate for each hospital is display as a point on a vertical line. These lines represent the amount of random variation in the NICU mortality rate data for that site.

1. Find medical literature references to identify patient factors associated with death of an infant in NICU. These factors were most likely used to risk-adjust the mortality data shown in figures B.2 and B.3.

2. Write a report that includes the following information:

    a. Results of your research, or the patient factors that you found to be associated with infant death in NICU. Include the references you used.

    b. Explain why mortality rates are lower at all hospitals when the data are risk-adjusted.

    c. Speculate as to why the mortality rate at some hospitals is still high when compared to others, even when the data are risk-adjusted.

Figure B.2: Risk-adjusted NICU mortality data

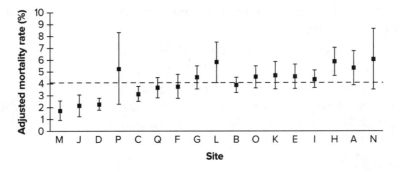

Figure B.3: Crude (not risk-adjusted) NICU mortality data

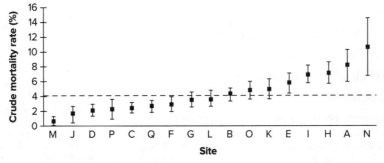

Source for Figures B.2 and B.3: Sankaran K, Chien LY, Walker R, Seshia M, and Ohlsson A, Canadian Neonatal Network. 2002. Variations in mortality rates among Canadian neonatal intensive care units. *CMAJ*. 166(2):173-8.

B.6 Recognize Use for Common Performance Improvement Tools

Description

Various performance improvement (PI) tools are used in an improvement project. In this project you'll identify common tools used during an improvement project and describe the purpose of the tools.

Instructions

1. Download the answer sheet for this project from the AHIMA student website.

2. Read the summary of the cardiovascular quality improvement case study that accompanies this project.

3. Using the answer sheet provided, indicate the PI tools that were used or could have been used during each project step. The PI tools are alluded to, but not specifically stated in the project description. Identify the tools are based on the description of how the tools were used during the step.

4. In addition to identifying the PI tools, also indicate what the tool helped the team accomplish.

Cardiovascular quality improvement case study

Step 1:   Identify Improvement Opportunity

The medical staff peer review process in a hospital cardiovascular service identified several instances of bleeding following percutaneous transluminal coronary angioplasty (PTCA) and cardiac catheterization procedures. A study was done to determine the extent of the problem. Of the 100 patient charts retrospectively reviewed, 14 (14%) had some bleeding, ranging from minor to severe. PTCA and cardiac catheterizations were reported separately, as follows:

> 88 Cath patients, 9 had some bleeding difficulties (10%)
> 12 PTCA patients, 5 had some bleeding difficulties (42%).

The issue was referred to the quality council, where leadership recommended the formation of a quality improvement team to investigate the process of care for patient undergoing PTCA and cardiac catheterization. The team was charged with identifying ways to improve the process and to decrease post-procedure bleeding problems.

Step 2:   Organize a Team

The following people served on the team:

- 2 interventional cardiologists who are members of the intraoperative cardiac team
- 1 cardiac surgeon
- 2 floor nurses involved with post-procedure care
- Cardiovascular services medical director
- Cardiovascular services administrative director
- Cardiovascular case manager
- Data analyst from quality management department

One cardiologist and the case manager served as the co-leaders of the team.

Step 3:   Gather Information

At the first team meeting, the group decided that they needed to validate the earlier study findings. A concurrent study was done, this time focusing on PTCA patients but also to verify the findings about cardiac catheterization patients from the first study. The team designed a data collection tool that was to be completed by the people directly involved with patient care following the procedure. The physicians developed criteria for reporting the amount of bleeding. It was agreed that the parameters and approach needed to be consistent for all patients studied.

The first section of the form was to be completed by the nurse assigned to the patient immediately following the procedure. The second section was to be completed by the nurse four hours following the procedure (the intent was for this to be the same person) and the last section was to be completed by the physician as he or she evaluated the incision site prior to discharge. Patients who did have bleeding would be ranked as to whether bleeding was minor, moderate, or severe (as defined by the criteria developed by physicians). The team decided that data would be gathered for the next 100 consecutive patients that underwent cardiac catheterization and/or PTCA. Data were gathered and the results shown below:

55 PTCA patients, 11 had bleeding difficulties (20%)
100 Cath patients, 9 had bleeding difficulties (9%).

The next team meetings were devoted to analyzing the issues and determining the most probable causes of the bleeding problems. The team used several PI tools to analyze the process of patient care (starting with the preoperative phase), narrow down the list of possible causes, and to determine the variables and probable reasons for post-operative bleeding problems.

Step 4:   Select Actions
The data collected in Step 3 and the PI tools helped the team identify the origin of bleeding problems. The team agreed that not all variables impacting patient outcomes could be eliminated, especially those related to patient characteristics. A PI tool was used to judge the advantages and disadvantages of each proposed action plan. Ultimately the team selected the following three process changes:

1. Reduce the size of the sheath used for angioplasty from a 9FR to an 8FR.
2. Stop heparin immediately after the PTCA procedure for all stable patients.
3. Remove the sheath within 4 hours following the procedure.

These changes were put into effect immediately with plans to pilot test the results.

Step 5:   Test the Effect
A follow-up study was done in one month to evaluate the effectiveness of the process changes. Of the 41 PTCA and Cath cases evaluated, 5 had bleeding difficulties (12%). The process changes appeared to have resulted in an 8% decrease in post-procedure bleeding. A review of patient outcomes (for example, reclosure and complication rates) confirmed that the changes made to the process did not compromise the quality of care.

Step 6:   Adopt the Change
The standard surgical set-up for PTCA and cardiac catheterization procedures was changed to include a smaller sheath (8FR). The process changes were incorporated into the clinical path for PTCA and cardiac catheterization patients and standard post-operative orders were changed to include an order for the technicians to pull sheaths 4 hours post-procedure.

Step 7:   Monitor Performance
A second follow-up survey in six months of 55 patients showed only 6 (11%) with bleeding difficulties. This represented an additional 1% decrease in bleeding since the pilot test. Additional follow-up studies were planned in 12 months to determine if the rate of post-procedure bleeding remains low.

B.7 Select PI Tools to Use During an Improvement Project

Description

Performance improvement (PI) tools are qualitative and quantitative tools used during an improvement project. The tools help advance the initiative toward achieving improvement goals. In this project, you'll pick which PI tool is best to use during different steps of an improvement initiative.

Background

Presume you are the supervisor of the patient records and billing department in a busy ophthalmology clinic. Staff and patient complaints about your department have been getting more frequent. Opticians complain they cannot quickly get patient's out-of-pocket cost estimates from the billing staff. Clinic receptionists are frustrated that staff in your department will not help cover the phones during breaks. Some patients have complained about delays in getting their records and on occasion a patient finds an error in the insurance billing. An ongoing problem has been long hold time when patients call with questions. You talk with staff in your department. They feel understaffed and cannot rely on clinic receptions to help with patient questions. Often phone calls are unnecessarily transferred by the receptionists to the records or billing staff. The medical assistants interrupt records staff to print clinic notes they could just as easily have printed themselves. Physicians are often unavailable to answer clinical questions necessary for coding and that delays billing. You need to improve teamwork among your department and other clinic staff and resolve the process problems. You decide to conduct an improvement project.

Instructions

1. Download the answer sheet for this project from the AHIMA student website.
2. Answer the following questions and record them on the answer sheet provided for this project.

   - What one performance improvement tool would you use to identify all possible reasons why complaints about your department are increasing? Briefly explain in your own words why this tool would be useful for this purpose.

   - What one performance improvement tool would you use to gather information to confirm the actual reasons for complaints about your department? Briefly explain in your own words why this tool would be useful for this purpose.

   - You think there may be more complaints on certain days of the week. What one performance improvement tool would you use to analyze this theory? Briefly explain in your own words why this tool would be useful for this purpose.

   - You tally information about types of complaints about your department. What one performance improvement tool would you use to select the complaints to eliminate first? Briefly explain in your own words why this tool would be useful for this purpose.

   - What one performance improvement tool would you use to understand the current process for obtaining information about patient's expected out-of-pocket costs for new glasses and communicating the information to opticians? Briefly explain in your own words why this tool would be useful for this purpose.

   - After redesigning the process for obtaining information about patient's expected out-of-pocket costs for new glasses and communicating the information to opticians, you want to monitor the effectiveness of your actions. What one performance improvement tool would you use to measure whether the number of complaints about delays decline over the next six months? Briefly explain in your own words why this tool would be useful for this purpose.

Tips: Keep the purpose of various PI tools in mind when completing the project – think about what is being done at each step and which tool is best for the job.

B.8   Improve Process Reliability

Description

Years of research in the design of interactive systems involving people, tools, and technology have resulted in an understanding of how best to optimize performance using human factors principles. In this project, you'll suggest ways of making a process more reliable using human factors principles.

There are seven basic human factors principles for making work system improvements:

- Simplify the process (take unnecessary steps out of the process)
- Standardize (remove variation and promote consistency)
- Reduce reliance on memory (provide tools such as checklists)
- Improve information access (make it easier to know what to do)
- Use constraints and forcing functions (make it less likely the task will be done incorrectly)
- Design for errors (create processes to prevent common mistakes)
- Adjust the environment (reduce the negative impact of surroundings)

Figure B.4 is a high-level flowchart of steps in the process of responding to external requests for copies of information from patient health records.

Figure B.4:   Process for releasing patient health records

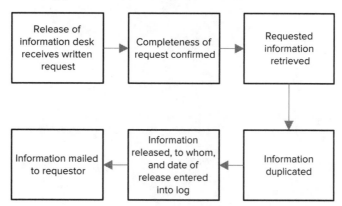

Instructions

Your task is to make the process more reliable to ensure the right information is released quickly after receipt of the request, the information is given to the right people, and facts about the release are accurately documented. Recommend at least three ways to improve the reliability of this process using the seven human factors principles listed in the description. Explain three changes you would make and which principle the change is based on.

References and Bibliography

Cantor, Michael D., Paul Barach, Arthur Derse, Claire W. Maklan, Ginger Schafer Wlody, Ellen Fox. 2005. "Disclosing adverse events to patients." *The Joint Commission Journal on Quality and Patient Safety* 31, (January): 5-12. https://doi.org/10.1016/s1553-7250(05)31002-6.

Center for Medicare and Medicaid Services (CMS). 2014. "Medicare ESRD Network Organizations: Glossary." https://www.cms.gov/Regulations-and-Guidance/Guidance/Manuals/downloads/eno114glossary.pdf.

Centers for Medicare and Medicaid Services (CMS). 2021. "HCAHPS: Patients' Perspectives of Care Survey." https://www.cms.gov/Medicare/Quality-Initiatives-Patient-Assessment-Instruments/HospitalQualityInits/HospitalHCAHPS.

Centers for Medicare and Medicaid Services (CMS). 2023. "Hospital Measures and Update Frequency." https://data.cms.gov/provider-data/topics/hospitals/measures-and-current-data-collection-periods.

Jabour, Abdulrahman M., Brian E. Dixon, Josette F. Jones, David A. Haggstrom. 2018. "Toward Timely Data for Cancer Research: Assessment and Reengineering of the Cancer Reporting Process." *JMIR Cancer*, 4, no. 1. http://doi.org/10.2196/cancer.7515.

Zimmer, Christian, Markus Norbert Janssen, Tanja Astrid Treschan, Jürgen Peters. 2004. "Near-miss Accident during Magnetic Resonance Imaging by a 'Flying Sevoflurane Vaporizer' due to Ferromagnetism Undetectable by Handheld Magnet." *Anesthesiology* 100, no. 5 (May): 1329–1330. https://doi.org/10.1097/00000542-200405000-00054.